DISEASES and DISORDERS
of the PIG

A Colour Atlas of
DISEASES and DISORDERS
of the PIG

W.J. Smith
BVMS, MRCVS
Senior Veterinary Investigation Officer
Scottish Agricultural Colleges
Veterinary Investigation Centre
Mill of Craibstone
Bucksburn
Aberdeen
Scotland

D.J. Taylor
MA, PhD, VetMB, MRCVS
Senior Lecturer in Veterinary Microbiology
University of Glasgow Veterinary School
Bearsden Road
Bearsden
Glasgow
Scotland

Prof. R.H.C. Penny
DVSc, PhD, FRCVS, DPM
Nether End
Austrey
Nr Atherstone
Warwickshire

Wolfe Publishing Limited

Copyright © W.J. Smith, D.J. Taylor, R.H.C. Penny, 1990
Published by Wolfe Publishing Ltd, 1990
Printed by W.S. Cowell Ltd, Ipswich, England
ISBN 0 7234 0996 X

A CIP catalogue record for this book is available from the British Library.

This book is one of the titles in the series of Wolfe Atlases, a series that
brings together the world's largest systematic published collection of
diagnostic colour photographs.

For a full list of Atlases in the series, plus forthcoming titles and details
of our veterinary Atlases, please write to Wolfe Publishing Ltd,
2-16 Torrington Place, London WC1E 7LT, England.

Contents

Preface

Although there are liberally illustrated books on pig diseases in other languages, this Colour Atlas is the first publication in English on the subject in which illustrations take precedence over the text.

The nature of the skin of most pigs (particularly the White breeds) means that it lends itself easily to photographic illustration, because any change from the norm is immediately obvious. Furthermore, the way the pig responds to its environment, to management and disease, can also be captured on film.

Limitations of space have forced the authors to concentrate on the more serious and common conditions, although single illustrations of some of the rarer pig diseases have been included wherever possible. The authors have deliberately excluded photomicrographs, illustrations of bacteria etc., since the emphasis of this book is on practical observation rather than laboratory techniques, and texts on laboratory diagnosis are readily available.

The subject matter covered includes not only the classic infectious diseases, but also highlights some disorders of multifactorial aetiology where the cause is of a more complex nature. Because of this there is, inevitably, some degree of overlap in subject matter between chapters. Where appropriate, the attention of the reader is drawn to other areas of the text which may be relevant.

The overriding aim of the authors was to produce a book in which the illustrations, used in conjunction with a standard textbook on pig diseases, would help to establish a diagnosis. An accurate diagnosis benefits both the pig and the farmer. This Atlas will be of help not only to the veterinarian and veterinary students, but also to the pig farmer, head stockman, meat inspector and others worldwide who are concerned with the health and management of pigs.

Acknowledgements

The resources of the three authors, even with their varied experience, could not produce all the illustrations needed. They have begged and borrowed material from many friends and colleagues, and it is hoped that all of them have been thanked. These slides, and their donors, are listed below:

Crown copyright CVL (c): **2, 3, 11, 13, 17, 19, 22, 25, 27, 29, 35, 40, 41, 46, 47, 65, 69, 70, 71, 74, 75, 88, 91, 92, 93, 101, 107, 108, 113, 115, 116, 143, 209, 210, 222, 223, 224, 244, 245, 246, 256, 258, 259, 261, 264, 271, 272, 305, 312, 313, 349, 350, 351, 391, 406, 418, 419, 437, 488, 490, 509, 510, 551, 552, 576, 584, 599, 618, 635**

Dr W. Beesley: **225**
Mr R.D.A. Cameron: **255**
Allison Clark: **677, 678**
Prof. M. Clarkson: **216**
Dr G. Elliott: **640**
Dr C. Glossop: **636, 637, 638, 639**
Dr I. Herbert: **221, 236**
Dr A. Hogg: **523**
Mr A. Hunter: **109, 352, 353, 424, 438, 513**
Mr M. Jeffrey: **240, 241, 629, 630**
Prof. J.E.T. Jones: **269, 308, 309, 310, 311, 364, 365, 432**

Mr N. Kavanagh: **123**
Dr G. Lawson: **390, 392**
Dr Lincarovic: **247**
Dr K. Linklater: **114**
Mr J. Lund: **141, 142**
Mr E.A. McPherson: **253**
Merck Sharp and Dohme Ltd: **208, 233, 234**
Dr S.W. Michna: **366, 367, 372, 373, 374**
Mr B. Peet: **24**
Mr G. Pritchard: **443, 444, 445, 446, 447**
Dr L. Roberts: **10, 12, 239, 242, 282, 292, 322**
Dr L. Sidoli and Dr E. Barigazzi: **439–441**
Prof. E.L. Soulsby: **217, 218**
Mr B. Spence: **273, 274, 275**
Dr J. Thomson; **129, 306, 524, 643, 644**
U.S. Department of Agriculture: **499–505**
Dr P. Whittlestone: **425–427**
Mr N. Wood: **453–460, 529**

Our grateful thanks are due to Mrs Diane Stuart, who typed the manuscript.

Finally, the authors would like to thank the publishers for their help and encouragement during the preparation of this Atlas.

Abnormalities, Hereditary and Developmental

Abnormalities may be developmental (environmental) or genetic in origin. Both may or may not be congenital (present at birth). Developmental abnormalities may be due to physical, chemical or infectious factors (teratogens). For example, excessive heat during a specific stage of foetal development, chemicals from poisonous plants such as hemlock, and uterine infections with viruses such as Swine Fever may cause these abnormalities.

Genetic defects are usually inherited, but may also arise due to mutations within the gametes or to chromosomal aberrations. Once genetic defects arise, they usually become heritable but as with many inherited conditions, the embryo or foetus often dies.

Developmental and genetic disorders must ultimately operate through common pathways, so it is not surprising that similar abnormalities may have different causes, (phenocopies). Cleft palate, for instance, may be inherited in a simple Mendelian fashion or may arise from a teratogenic effect, as in Vitamin A deficiency. The absolute cause of many abnormalities is not known and many disorders apparently inherited in a complex fashion, have a strong environmental component *e.g.* atresia ani.

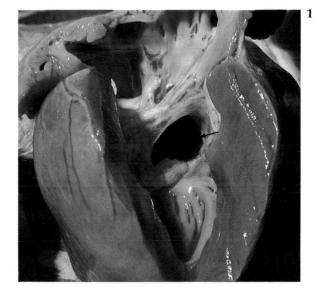

1 Interventricular septal defect or 'hole in the heart' in a 15 kg pig. Cause unknown. The defect is marked with an arrow.

Iso-immunisation

Iso-immunisation of pregnancy is a genetically dependent phenomenon which arises when incompatible foetal blood antigens cross the placental barrier. The dam becomes immunised against the incompatible cells and the iso-antibodies reach future piglets via colostrum. Haemolytic disease occurs if the iso-antibodies are directed against red blood cells (**2**) while if directed against platelets thrombocytopenic purpura will ensue (**3**). This may also occur following use of vaccines containing blood, such as Crystal Violet Swine Fever Vaccine.

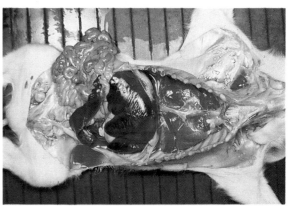

2 Haemolytic disease A three-day-old piglet with pale musculature and watery blood.

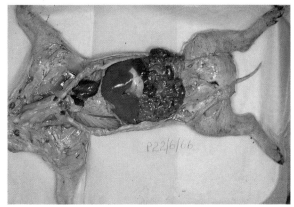

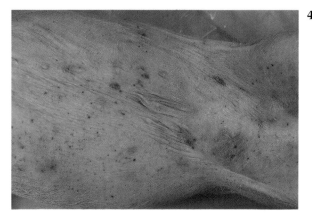

3 Thrombocytopenic purpura A six-day-old piglet. Note the pale carcase and widespread petechial haemorrhages in the skin, bladder and gut. All lymph nodes have a haemorrhagic appearance.

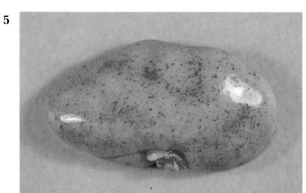

4 Thrombocytopenic purpura A four-day-old piglet. Close-up of skin haemorrhages in the ventral abdomen.

5 Kidney from the piglet in **4** note the widespread petechial haemorrhages.

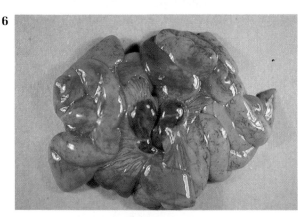

6 Thrombocytopenic purpura The small intestine of the piglet in **4**. Note the haemorrhages in the gut wall and the haemorrhagic lymph nodes.

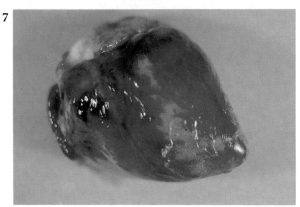

7 Thrombocytopenic purpura The heart from the piglet in **4**.

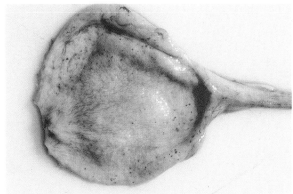

8

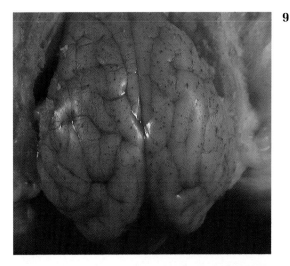

9

8 Thrombocytopenic purpura Bladder mucosa from the piglet **4**. Note the petechial haemorrhages on the mucosa.

9 Thrombocytopenic purpura Brain haemorrhages.

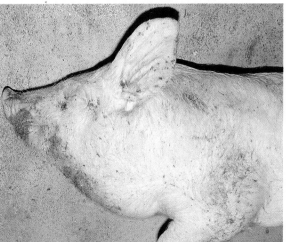

10

10 Lymphosarcoma Lymphosarcoma may be an inherited disease in the pig (autosomal recessive in the Large White). Note the swelling of the neck and entrance to the chest due to massive swelling of the thymus. Where submandibular swelling is observed in a finishing pig, lymphosarcoma should be suspected.

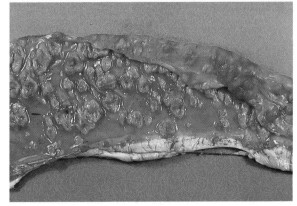

11

11 Lymphosarcoma Small intestine. These raised lesions are usually accompanied by lymphatic lesions elsewhere in the carcase.

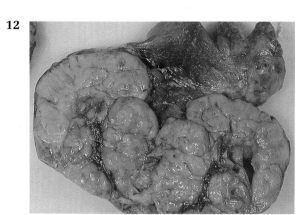 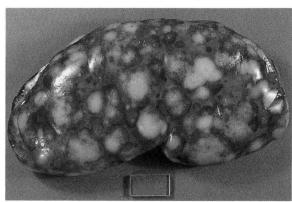

12 Lymphosarcoma of the thymus (*see* **10**).

13 Lymphosarcoma Kidney.

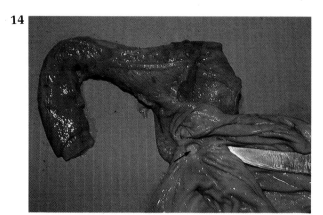 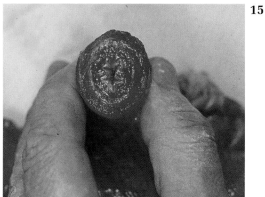

14 Oesophageal muscular hypertrophy in a 20 kg weaner. Note the absence of the pars oesophagea. The arrow points to the oesophageal entrance. The point of the knife lies in the diverticulum.

15 Cross-section of the oesophagus of the animal in **14**. The thickening is associated with diffuse hypertrophy of muscularis mucosa, particularly involving circumferential muscle layers. There was no abnormality of serosa or mucosa.

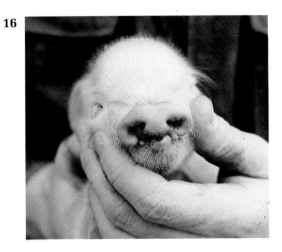

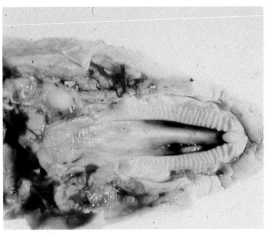

16 and **17 Cleft palate** Pigs are born alive but the extent of the lesion makes sucking difficult and affected animals usually die. Sometimes the condition may be suspected without having to examine the palate as in **16**. The lesions may be inherited or developmental in origin.

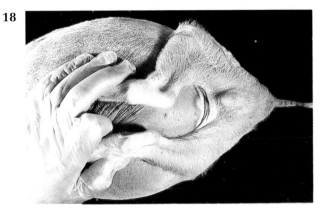

18 Atresia ani in a male piglet.

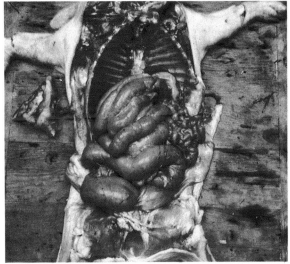

19 Atresia ani Note the dilated colon. Affected pigs normally die between 10 days and three weeks of age. In females the rectal contents may burst into the vagina to give a recto-vaginal fistula and allow survival to adulthood.

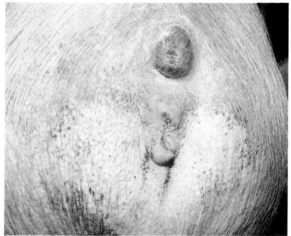

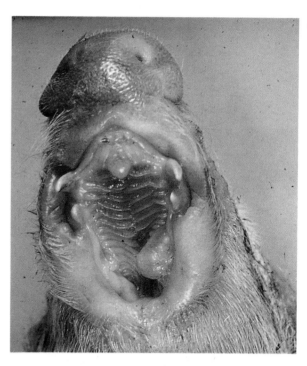

20 Recto-vaginal fistula This two-year-old
sow had conceived twice and was pregnant for
the third time when this photograph was taken
(*see* **19**).

21 Agnathia Absence of the lower jaw, cause
unknown.

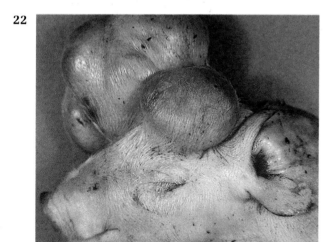

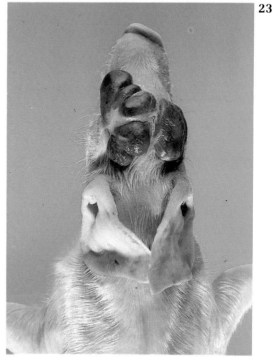

22 and **23 Meningoencephalocele** Normally
pigs with this condition die at birth. These are
typical cases. The condition results from
failure of fusion of the frontal bones during
development.

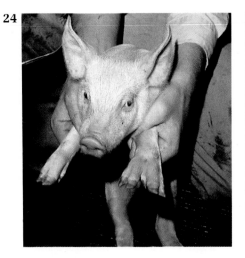

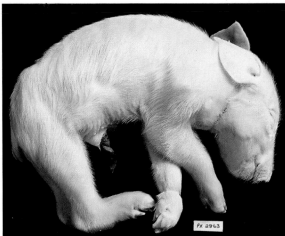

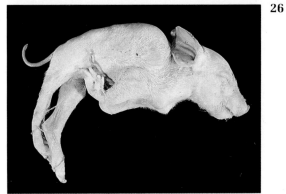

24 **Polydactyly** affecting the left forelimb only. Pigs may survive to slaughter with this condition.

25 **Arthrogryposis** This condition results in fixation of the joints and may be due to a number of different causes but is frequently teratogenic in origin.

26 **Arthrogryposis and kyphosis** A stillborn piglet.

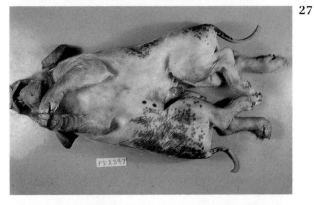

27 **Siamese twins**.

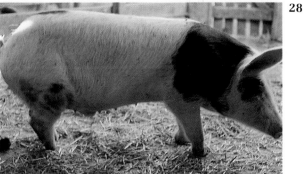

28 **Amputate** Complete absence of digits.

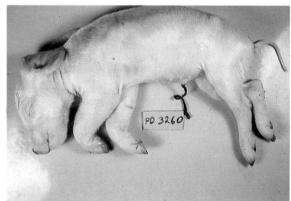

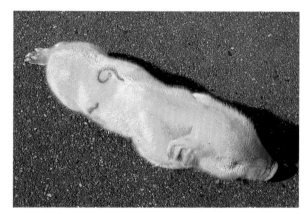

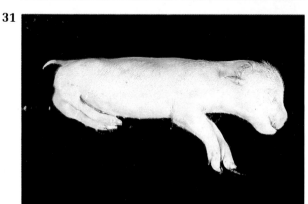

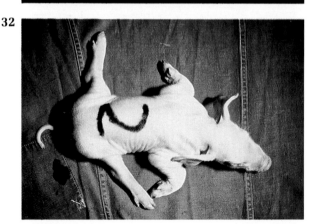

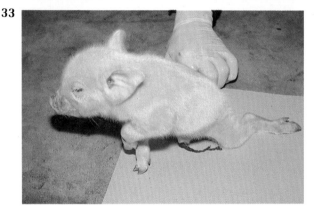

29 Thickleg (hyperostosis) This congenital condition is always fatal. The radius and ulna of both front legs are always enlarged, hard and do not pit on pressure (*see* **96**).

30 Congenital hemimelia This live two-day-old piglet has no tibia and cannot stand. Varying degrees of tibial hypoplasia occurred in the litter.

31 Congenital hemimelia A stillborn piglet with complete absence of tibia.

32 Splayleg In this case all four legs are affected. If piglets are able to suckle, or are fed artificially, they will become clinically normal within two to four days and survive. The condition is more common in the Landrace breed.

33 Atypical 'splayleg' of the hindlegs This condition has been noted in the offspring of hybrid gilts mated to Large White boars. Some piglets may be born affected, while others develop the disorder within three days of birth. The condition presents as an inability of the piglet to use its hind legs correctly so that it often assumes a dog-sitting position with both hind legs extended alongside the body and not laterally as in true splayleg. The front legs never splay but do seem to have a spastic, jerky movement occasionally when the piglet walks. Attempts to rise and walk usually end in the hind legs sliding underneath the piglet in extension.

Affected piglets do not recover in three-four days as with true splayleg and mortality is high. Deep pain withdrawal reflexes and hind limb placing reflexes are poor. Histopathological examination suggested a mild sub-acute axonpathy of spinal cord and brain stem (cause unknown).

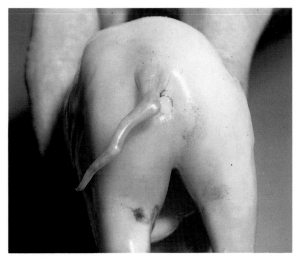

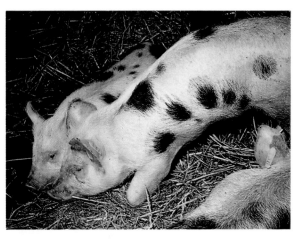

34 Kinky tail (congenital) A common condition of pigs.

35 Pietrain creeper syndrome This is a non-congenital familial disease of progressive muscular weakness beginning at three weeks of age and ending in permanent recumbency at approximately 12 weeks of age. It is characterised by progressive myodegeneration and atrophy with fibrosis and fatty replacement.

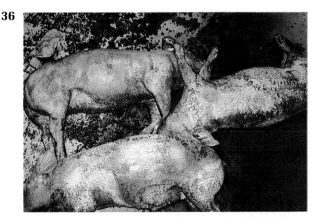

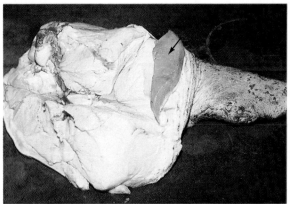

36 Porcine Stress Syndrome (PSS) – transport deaths All three pigs died on the same lorry en route to the abattoir. Pigs of certain breeds *eg.*, Pietrain, Landrace, are particularly susceptible to stress and are liable to die. Clinical signs include tremors of muscle and tail, marked dyspnoea, patchy erythema, cyanosis, hyperthermia and muscle rigidity. Post mortem signs vary greatly but often include patchy skin cyanosis, paleness of some muscle groups and evidence of heart/lung failure such as generalised oedema of the lungs and an excessive frothy exudate in the bronchi and trachea.

37 Porcine Stress Syndrome The hind leg of an 85 kg pig, a sudden death case. Note the pale soft, exudative (PSE) muscle with a normal portion of muscle (arrow) from the same pig overlain for comparison.

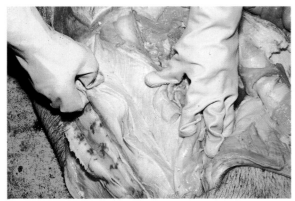

38 Porcine Stress Syndrome Note the pale longissimus dorsi muscle.

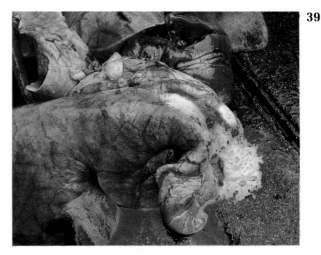

39 Porcine Stress Syndrome Lungs from the pig in **37**. Note the generalised oedema, congestion of lungs and frothy exudate from the trachea.

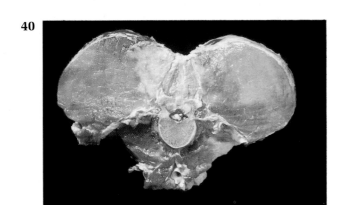

40 Porcine Stress Syndrome Back Muscle Necrosis (BMN). Note the pale areas of necrosis in the multifidi and longissimus dorsi muscles.

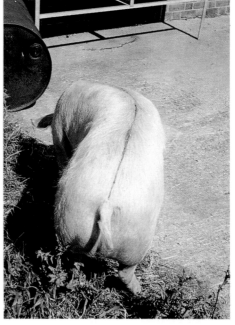

41 Porcine Stress Syndrome Back Muscle Necrosis. This is a special manifestation of the porcine stress syndrome in animals over 50kg. In unilateral cases in live animals there is curvature of the body towards the affected side.

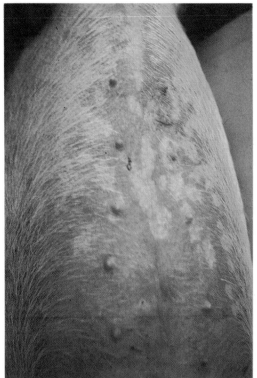

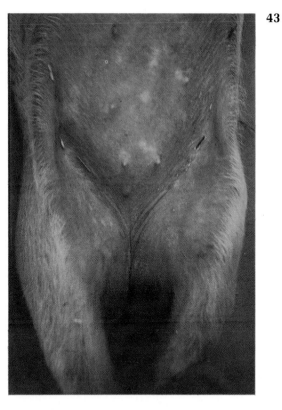

42 Porcine Stress Syndrome A proportion of modern, hybrid pigs show lesions of erythema when restrained. If not released quite rapidly they may die. This·condition is probably associated with stress susceptibility and PSE.

43 Porcine Stress Syndrome A more severe reaction than shown in **42**.

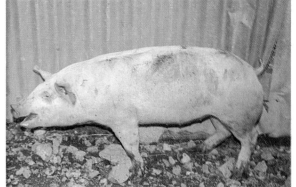

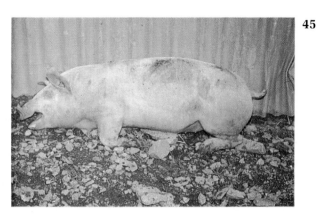

44 Porcine Stress Syndrome As this 65 kg pig was being moved to another house it became severely distressed and collapsed.

45 Porcine Stress Syndrome The same pig as in **44**, 40 seconds before death occurred. Post mortem confirmed PSS.

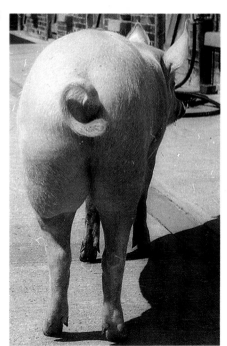

46 Asymmetric Hindquarter Syndrome Note the volumetric asymmetry of the hindquarters. This disorder of finishing pigs may arise spontaneously and then subside on its own.

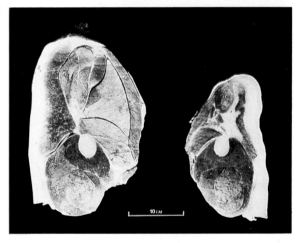

47 Asymmetric Hindquarter Syndrome Mid-femur section of the thighs from the pig in **46**. Note the increased subcutaneous fat on the larger side and the reduced muscle volume on the smaller side.

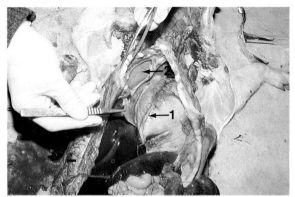

48 Congenital diaphragmatic hernia in a four-week-old pig. Note how the stomach (1) lies in the left pleural cavity while the heart (2) is pushed to the right. The remains of the diaphragm are held by the lower forceps. Death was eventually due to heart and lung failure.

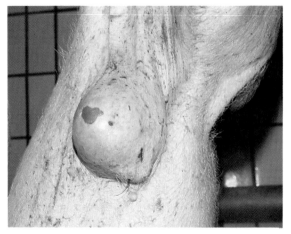

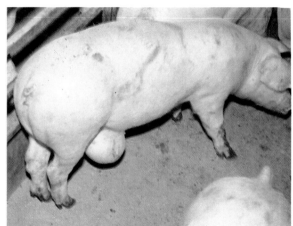

49–51 Umbilical hernia Occasionally the intestines may become incarcerated in the hernia, leading to intestinal obstruction and death (*see* **618**). These are typical cases of umbilical hernia.

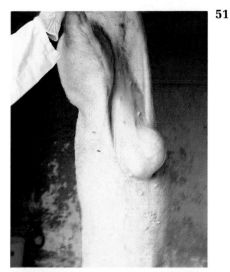

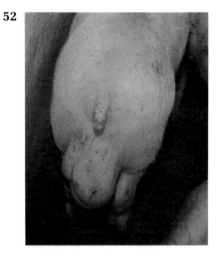

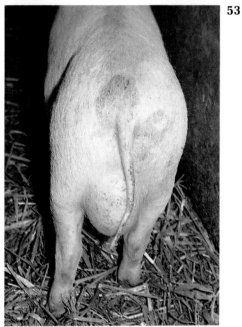

52 and **53 Scrotal hernia** This condition may be present at birth but frequently does not become obvious until the pig is at least six weeks old. These are typical unilateral cases.

54

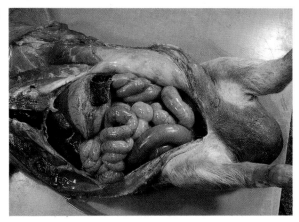

54 Scrotal hernia This scrotal hernia has become strangulated and the pig died from the consequences. The bowel loop was trapped by fibrinous and fibrous adhesions and became necrotic. Note the discoloured skin over the hernia.

55

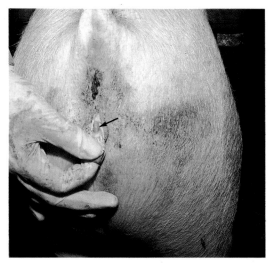

55 Male pseudohermaphrodite (genetically female) Note the enlarged clitoris (arrow). Male gonads were present in this gilt but the rest of the reproductive tract had mainly female characteristics.

56

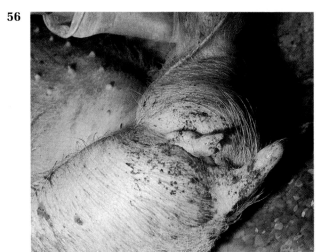

56 True hermaphrodite Masculinisation of the vulva; an upward-pointing 'tipped vulva' reflects abnormalities in the reproductive organs. The extent of the masculinisation varies from little or none to almost complete penis formation.

57 True hermaphrodite Reproductive organs from the pig shown in **56** The structure on the left is an ovary with an underdeveloped uterine horn and fallopian tube. The structure on the right is an ovarotestis with both vas deferens and vestigial uterine horn.

58 True hermaphrodite One ovary and one testicle. This gilt may breed but will produce a small litter. The uterus is normal.

57

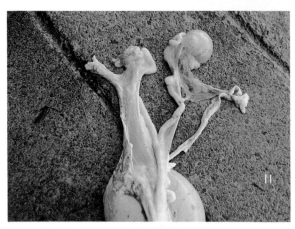

58

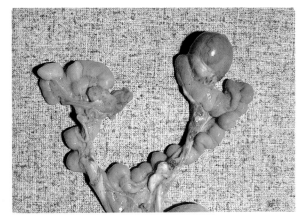

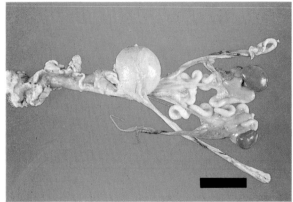

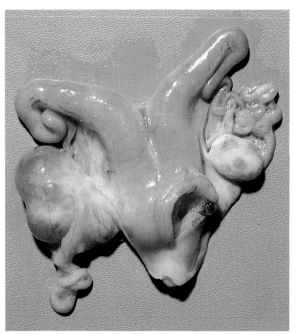

59 True hermaphrodite Ovarotestes with vestigial uterine horns arranged centrally. The two lateral structures are vasa deferentia not connected to the ovarotestes.

60 True hermaphrodite Ovarian and testicular tissue is present in one ovary. The uterus is grossly abnormal.

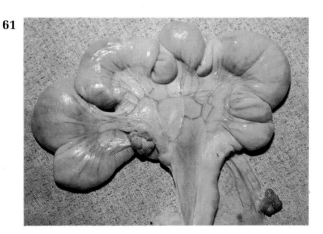

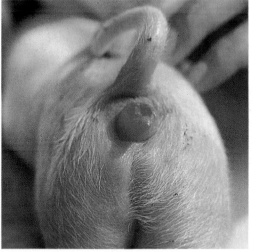

61 Uterus Unicornis Note the presence of two ovaries.

62 Congenital oedema of the vulva Piglets may be born with enlarged oedematous and congested vulvas in response to high levels of oestrogen in the dam. There are also other causes (*see* **247**).

63

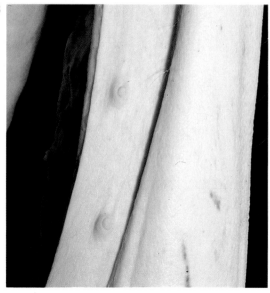

64

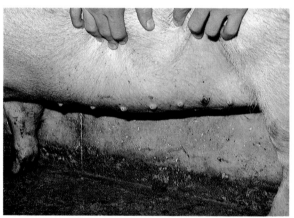

64 True inverted nipples in a gilt This may be a hereditary condition and there is no cure.

63 Pseudo inverted nipples this may be a hereditary condition but nipples will develop, erect and milk on farrowing.

65

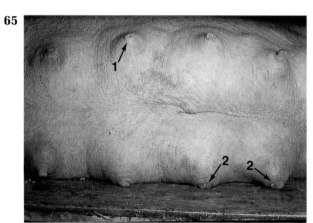

66

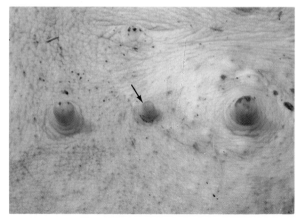

65 True and false inverted nipples Note the crater-like shape of the true inverted nipple (arrow 1). Such a nipple cannot be sucked. Two pseudo-inverted nipples are seen in the lower row (arrows 2).

66 Accessory nipple (arrow) on a 1st-litter gilt.

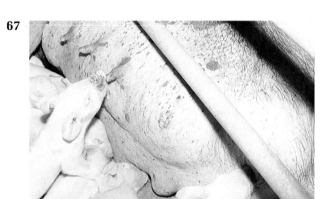

67 Nipple aplasia Note the complete absence of two nipples.

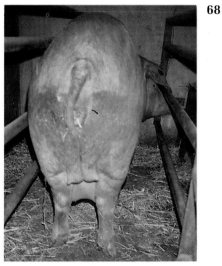

68 Supernumerary teats A sow in lactation.

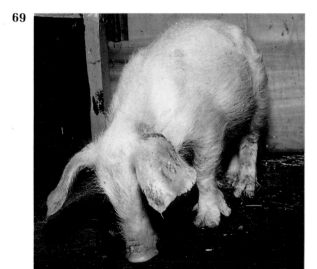

69–71 Dermatosis vegetans This is an inherited condition of Landrace pigs and is mainly characterised by skin lesions. Affected pigs die with a giant-cell pneumonia when five–six weeks old. Note the lesions on the skin of the shoulders (**70**) and feet (**71**).

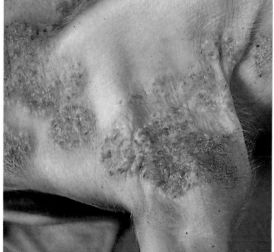

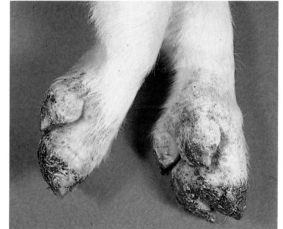

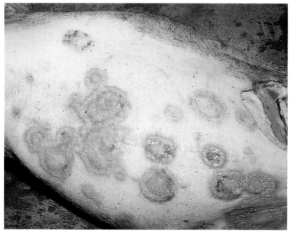

72

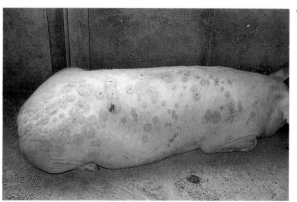

73

73 Atypical pityriasis rosea in a 10-month-old gilt.

72 Pityriasis rosea (pseudo ringworm) This condition appears at about 8–14 weeks of age and usually resolves within 10 weeks. It may, therefore, still be present at slaughter.

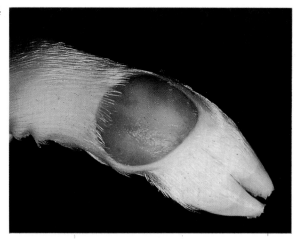

74

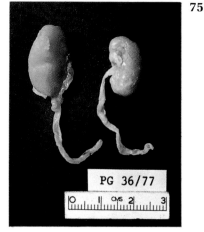

75

PG 36/77

74 Epitheliogenesis imperfecta The name is descriptive of the lesion. Such lesions can occur elsewhere on the body and in severe cases the piglets die.

75 Hypoplastic kidneys

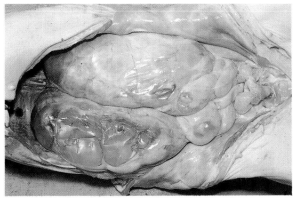

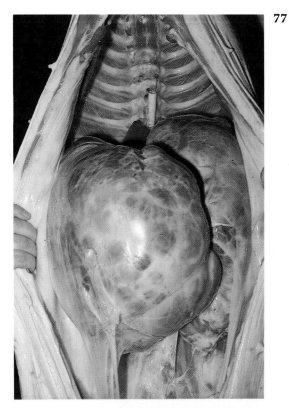

76 and **77** **Polycystic kidneys** in 70 kg pigs at
slaughter. These carcases were totally
condemned.

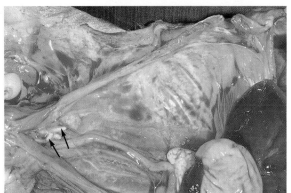

78 **Renal agenesis** in a two-day-old piglet
Complete absence of kidneys. The ureters
(arrows) are capped by metanephric tissue but
there is no kidney. Urates are present in the
body wall.

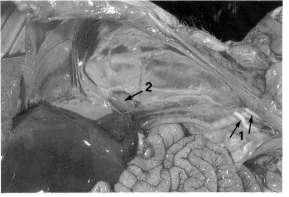

79 **Renal agenesis** a two-day-old piglet
showing ureters (1) and the adrenal gland (2)
in its normal position. The kidney has not
developed.

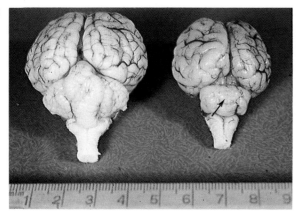

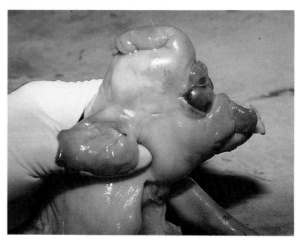

80 Cerebellar hypoplasia The cerebellum on the right (arrow) is affected. This condition may be due to foetal infection with some strains of swine fever virus, and also other viruses.

81 Cyclopia Cause unknown.

Nutritional Disorders

Nutritional diseases may be associated with an absolute deficiency of the nutrient concerned, as for example starvation or a deficiency of an essential nutrient (*e.g.* Vitamins A, D and E). They may also be conditioned deficiencies in which the mineral is present in the diet but cannot be absorbed because of the presence of substances which interfere with it. The uptake of calcium is particularly affected. It may be in an unavailable form or may be bound by substances such as phytate.

In other situations, nutrient levels may be adequate for maintenance but inadequate for growth, as in iron deficiency anaemia or zinc deficiency. Loss of nutrients in diarrhoea or zinc deficiency, particularly in the lactating sow (which requires calcium and energy), may also result in deficiency states.

Excess of nutrients or abnormal substances may lead to poisoning. Many nutritional conditions develop gradually and are restricted to animals maintained upon a single batch of feed (concentrate or grain) which lacks the nutrient concerned or contains too much of normal or poisonous substances.

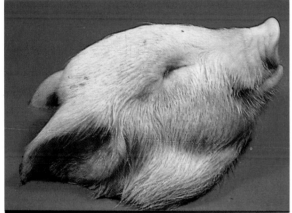

82 Vitamin A deficiency Micropthalmia due to dysmorphogenesis during the early part of gestation.

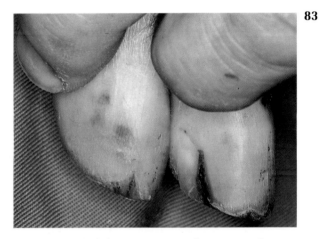

83 Biotin deficiency Haemorrhages into the horn of the wall are said to be common with this disease but they can readily be produced by trauma. Note the wall cracks.

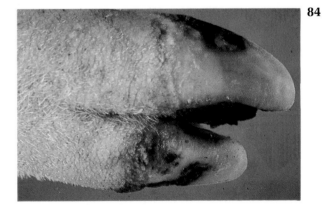

84 Biotin deficiency, experimentally induced. Note the wall and coronary band lesions.

85

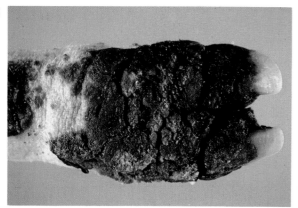

85 Biotin deficiency, experimentally induced and of long standing. Note the hyperkeratinisation of claws and skin.

Vitamin E – Selenium Deficiency

Deficiency of the above nutrients may produce characteristic yet overlapping lesions hence the use of several terms to describe different manifestations of the same complex – Mulberry Heart Disease; Hepatosis Dietetica; Nutritional Muscular Dystrophy; Dietetic Micro-angiopathy; Yellow Fat Disease; Hertzod.

Vitamin E maintains the integrity of the cell by preventing the oxidation of unsaturated lipid materials in cells to lipid hydroperoxides which can cause a variety of cell tissue damage. Selenium is involved in enzyme complexes which remove excess hydroperoxide. Mulberry Heart Disease is now common and may be a reflection on the large number of diets containing high levels of fat premixes – especially unsaturated fats and fat in an active state of peroxidation.

Barley often originates from soils low in selenium and wet storage under propionic acid treatment may destroy Vitamin E. These two factors may also have contributed to the recent increase in Mulberry Heart Disease and associated conditions.

86

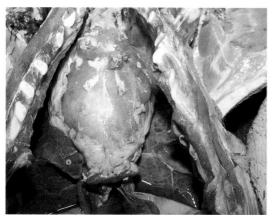

86 Mulberry Heart Disease The exposed chest cavity of a seven-week-old weaner. Note the pericardial sac bulging with fluid and the congested, oedematous lungs. The chest cavity always contains excessive straw-coloured fluid.

87

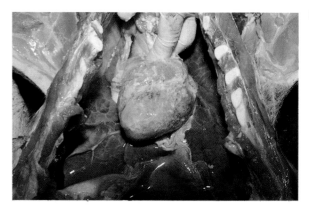

87 Mulberry Heart Disease The weaner in **86** showing the opened pericardial sac. Note the fibrinous desposits and myocardial haemorrhages.

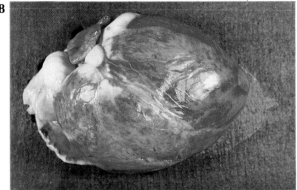

88 Mulberry Heart Disease Note the myocardial haemorrhages and dystrophic lesions (pale areas).

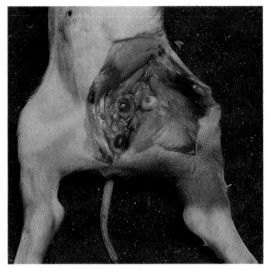

89 Vitamin E deficiency Piglets born to Vitamin E deficient dams are very susceptible to Iron Injection Toxaemia. Note the discoloration and thickening of the left leg due to oedema. (Compare the width of left and right tibia).

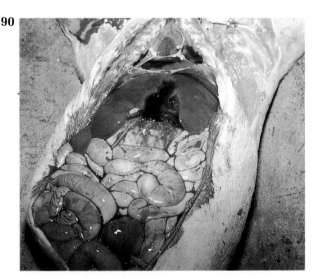

90 Vitamin E deficiency in a three-week-old piglet. Fatal haemorrhage from spontaneous rupture of the liver of 2–4 week-old piglets is not uncommon in suckling pigs and can often be the first indication of a Vitamin E-related problem.

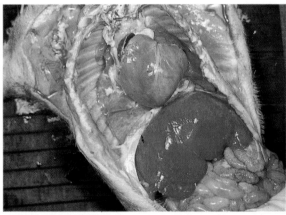

91 Iron deficiency anaemia Note the gross anaemia, characterised by a pale carcase, watery blood, enlarged heart and liver lesions. This deficiency is now rare but occasionally a pig may be missed by the stockperson when injecting iron.

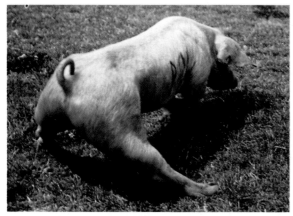

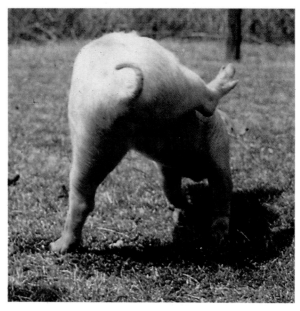

92 Pantothenic acid deficiency Pantothenic acid (a vitamin of the B complex) is involved in the metabolism and synthesis of fats, carbohydrates and proteins. Clinical signs of deficiency include inappetance, poor growth, diarrhoea, coughing and locomotor disturbances characterised by 'goose stepping'. The disorder is more prevalent in swill (garbage) fed pigs.

93 Pantothenic acid deficiency Note the 'goose stepping' gait.

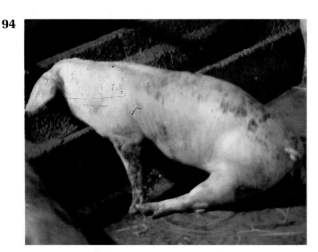

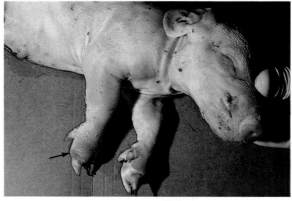

94 Pantothenic acid deficiency An affected swill-fed pig, 80kg, demonstrating the characteristic splay-legged posture. Goose-stepping was common amongst pigs which had been fed on boiled bakery waste.

95 Riboflavin deficiency Piglets born from dams with a deficiency of riboflavin may have congenital subcutaneous oedema of the forelegs – in this case especially above the claws of the forelegs (arrows).

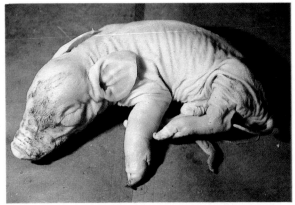

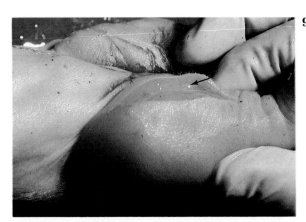

96 Riboflavin deficiency Newborn piglet with congenital subcutaneous oedema of the foreleg. This condition closely resembles thickleg (hyperostosis – *see* **29**).

97 Riboflavin deficiency The piglet from **96** with skin incised showing severe subcutaneous oedema (arrow).

98 Rickets Forelimb from a six-month-old stunted pig with severe rickets which rendered the animal ataxic. Note the enlarged carpus associated with pathological fractures. The length of the hair coat emphasises the stunting.

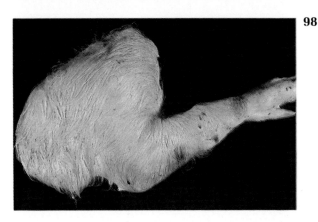

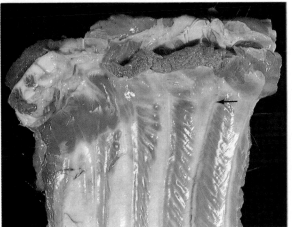

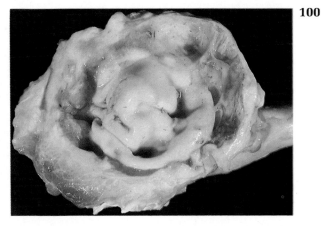

99 Rickets Swollen costochondral junctions (arrow) from the pig shown in **98**.

100 Rickets An enlarged shoulder joint, opened to reveal the collapsed cartilage.

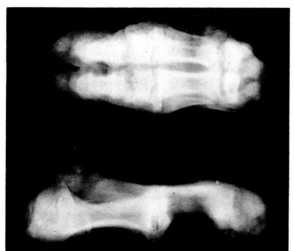

101 Rickets A radiograph of a forelimb showing typical bone lesions.

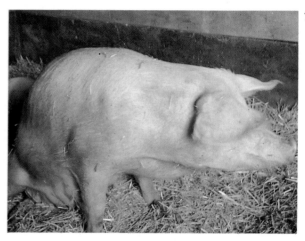

102 Osteomalacia in sows A modern hybrid gilt kept with a large eight-week litter was unable to rise. This animal recovered after the litter was weaned and parenteral calcium was given, confirming that the condition was associated with calcium deficiency. It has also been associated with lack of vitamin D in adult pigs.

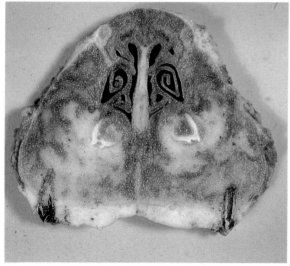

103 Osteodystrophia fibrosa (big head) This rare bone disease may result from (1) primary or secondary nutritional hyperparathyroidism, or (2) as a development of osteoporosis.

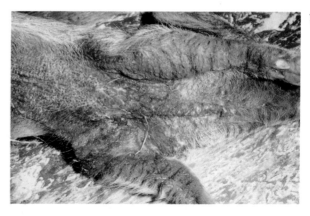

104 Parakeratosis Zinc deficiency results in symmetrical changes to the skin seen here on the carcase of a growing (25 kg) pig. It is most common in animals which are fed dry feed from the floor or from earthenware troughs and is rare where wet feeding or galvanised troughs are used. Diarrhoea may exacerbate the condition, as may excessive calcium or phytate in the diet.

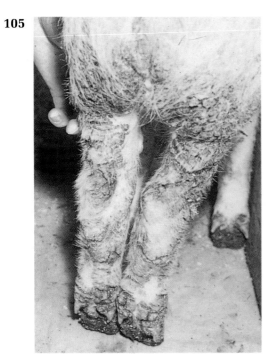

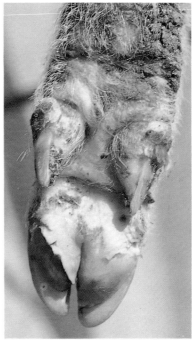

105 Parakeratosis A 14 kg weaner with typical lesions of parakeratosis. There is little or no skin irritation.

106 Parakeratosis lesions on the leg of 16 kg weaner.

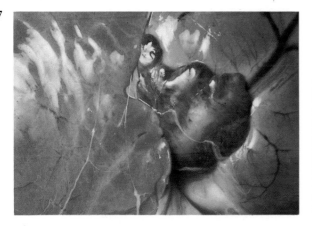

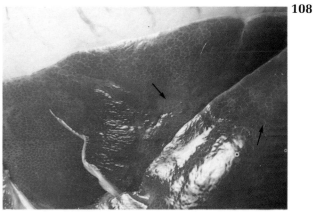

107 Bracken poisoning – heart and lung Bracken poisoning is an acquired thiamine deficiency resulting from the destruction of dietary thiamine by thiaminase found in bracken. The lesions are those of heart failure. Note the congestion and oedema of the lungs.

108 Bracken poisoning Lesions in the liver (arrows).

109

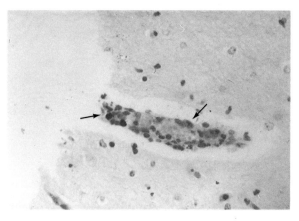

110

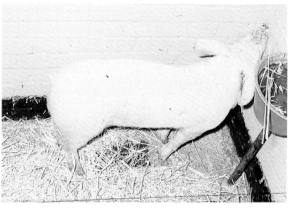

109 Salt poisoning or water deprivation
Eosinophils (arrows) can be seen around this
CNS blood vessel. This condition, also known
as sodium toxicosis, is very common and is
usually related to water deprivation rather than
high levels of salt, which pigs can tolerate well
providing they have access to plenty of water.
Clinically, the condition is characterised by
thirst, constipation, tonoclonic convulsions
and opisthotonus. Affected animals also appear
to be blind and deaf.

110 Salt poisoning or water deprivation
Weaner showing one of the typical signs of salt
poisoning, pressing of the head into a corner.

111

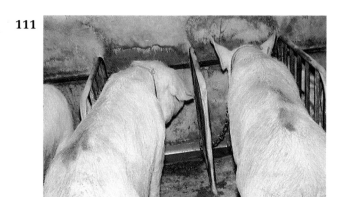

112

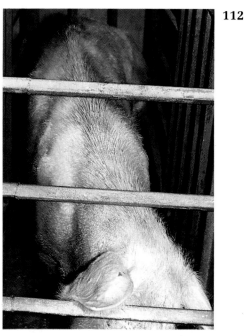

111 Thin Sows Although mainly a nutritional
deficiency this condition may be compounded
by the temperature of the environment and
other factors such as rearing large litters on a
low energy diet and parasitism. Once sows
have reached the state of pathological
emaciation they often die irrespective of the
quantity or quality of food given to them.

112 Thin sow This sow has reached the stage
of pathological emaciation and should be
culled.

13

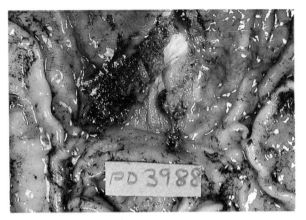

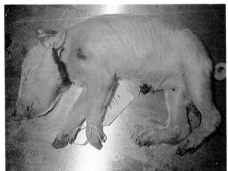

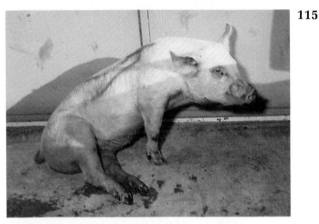

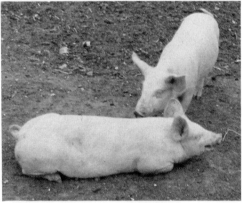

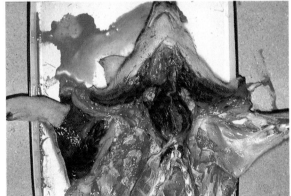

113 Copper poisoning Stomach showing haemorrhages, especially around the pars oesophagea. The inclusion of zinc at higher levels (110g/tonne) appears to prevent this condition which usually occurs when pigs are fed diets containing more than 220g/tonne copper sulphate.

114 Arthrogryposis due to hemlock (*Conium maculatum*) consumption by the dam. Tobacco may have a similar effect.

115 Haloxon poisoning/neurotoxicity Haloxon is an organophosphorus oral antihelminthic used in many species. This pig is showing posterior paralysis due to peripheral nerve degeneration – a typical symptom of delayed haloxon poisoning.

116 Poisoning from 3-Nitro-4-Hydroxy-phenylarsonic acid Live affected pigs with one in sternal recumbency and gasping. With this condition the skin of affected pigs may suddenly vary from normal in colour to an intense deep red colour, and then revert to normal. This usually occurs while the pig is having an attack of incoordination and ataxia.

117 Warfarin poisoning Note the extensive haemorrhages.

Management-related Disorders

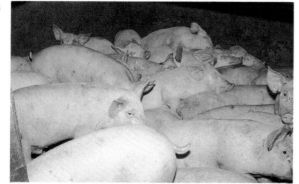

A large number and variety of conditions may arise from the confinement of pigs in intensive housing, or indeed in straw-bedded accommodation. These problems usually arise, not because of some inherent fault in the system but because of failure of management to run the system properly, maintain it at optimum functional level or, indeed, to construct it properly in the first instance.

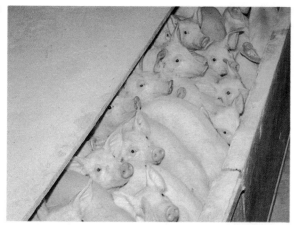

118 and **119** **Overcrowding.**

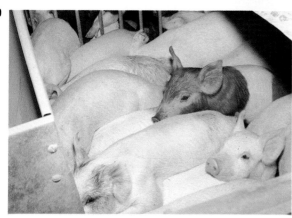

120 Lack of trough space This may lead to uneven growth rates and behavioural problems such as tail biting. (*see* **655).**

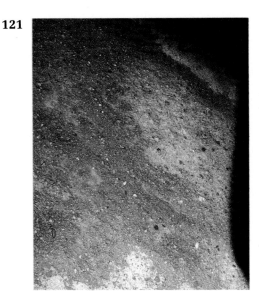

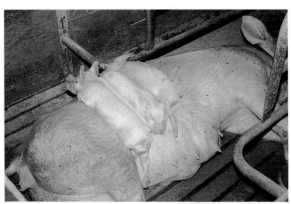

122 An unsuitable floor in farrowing pen
Note the preference of piglets for comfort.
These were the only piglets to survive out of a
litter of nine.

121 Concrete floor of a farrowing pen Note
the rough, abrasive surface due to exposure of
the aggregate – predisposing to damage of the
feet and legs of piglets.

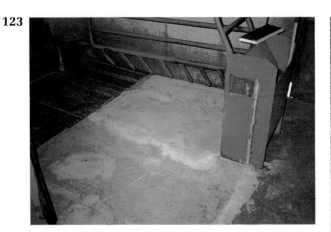

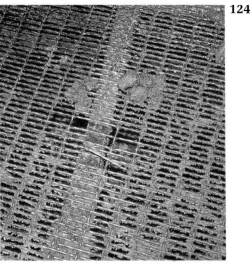

123 Unsuitable floor in a farrowing pen This
farrowing pen floor was resurfaced with a
special compound. Over-zealous use of a steel
float made it extremely slippery and resulted
in an increase in piglet mortality from 12% to
23%, due mainly to overlying.

**124 Woven wire mesh in a flat-deck weaner
pen** Note the fracture of the wire over the
support, resulting in sharp spikes liable to
injure pigs.

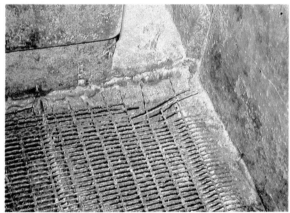

125 Woven wire panel fractured at the entrance to a pen. The sharp wire projections will almost certainly injure the pigs. Faulty laying was the cause in this instance.

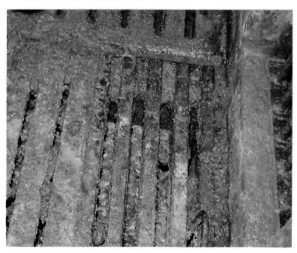

126 Unsuitable concrete slats in a finishing pen Note the narrow slats, wide gaps and rough edges – predisposing to claw damage.

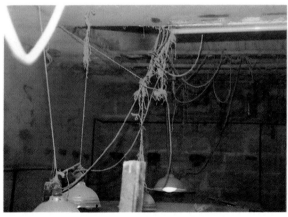

127 Example of poor workmanship in weaner pen An outbreak of fire or electrocution of either pigs or men is a likely possibility.

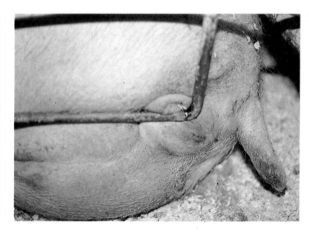

128 Sow due to farrow, confined in a farrowing crate. Note the retaining back bar pressing on the vulva. This may result in injury to the vulva *e.g.* haematoma (*see* 621).

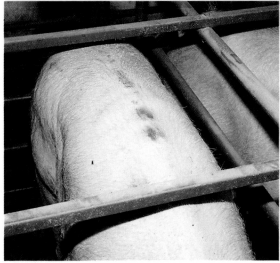

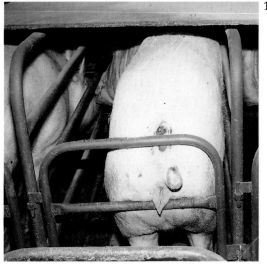

129 Sow stalls Note the damage to the sow's spine from a bar.

130 Sow stalls These sow stalls are too short. Note the pressure sore on the tail head.

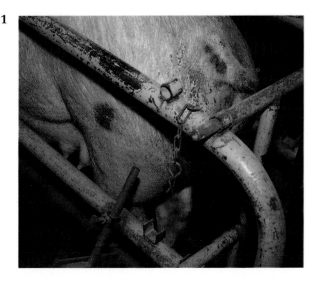

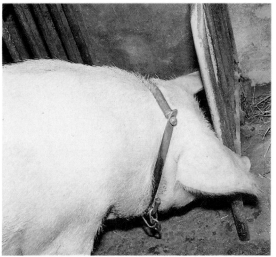

131 Sow in a farrowing crate Note the injury to the hip from a projecting anti-crush bar device.

132 Sow in a neck tether The tether is now too tight because of the rapid weight gain of the sow during pregnancy. Note that the tether is digging into the lower neck. Tethers need adjusting as the sow increases in condition, particularly in the first month.

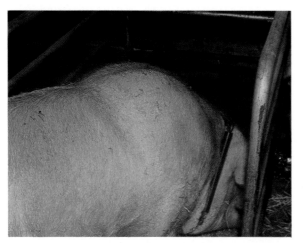

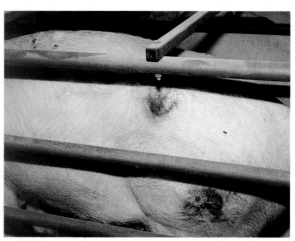

133 Neck-tethered sow This sow had been girth-tethered and, although the skin was not broken, this tether had caused some deformity of the back.

134 Sow in stall Note the pressure sores – a sequel to rapid loss of condition in a sow while suckling piglets on a perforated metal floor.

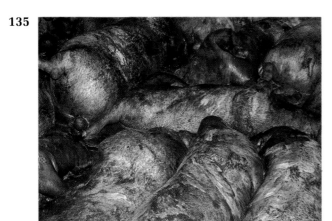

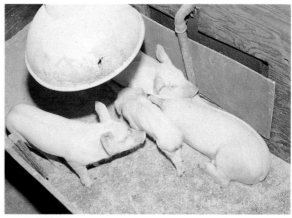

135 Hyperthermia Death of all pigs in a finishing pen due to hyperthermia after failure of the ventilation system. The photograph was taken approximately one and a half hours after death. Note the advanced state of decomposition.

136 Unthrifty weaner in a situation where it is unable to compete with larger pen mates. This pig should be placed in a pen with pigs of equal size or fostered back to a suitable lactating sow.

137 Unthrifty newly-weaned pigs requiring immediate removal to a hospital pen or back to a sow. These piglets had failed to recognise solid food, and consequently did not eat.

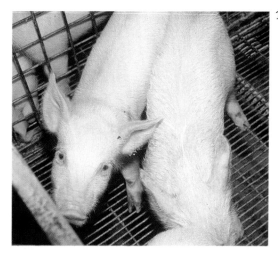

Abscesses

Abscesses may result from the use of contaminated needles or bottles containing contaminated vaccine or antibiotics. They may also occur as a result of fighting or castration. The most common site for abscessation is the neck or ham. Infection in the latter area results in considerable loss due to condemnation at slaughter. Normal hygienic precautions should prevent such problems arising. However, even sterile vaccines may provoke a reaction if the adjuvant is unsuitable. Pyaemia may also arise from skin wounds, especially those caused by fighting.

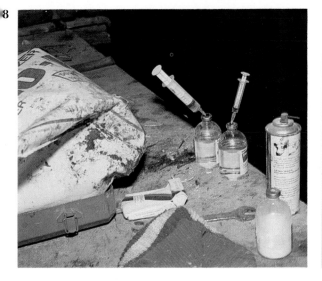

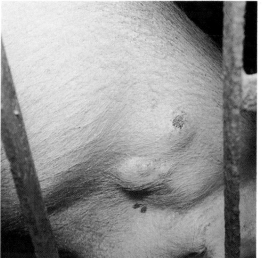

138 Unsuitable drug storage All drugs should be stored in a cool, dark cupboard or, when instructed, in a refrigerated cabinet. Sterile needles should be used at all times.

139 Abscess in the neck of a four-year-old sow – a common sequal to the use of a contaminated needle or faulty injection technique.

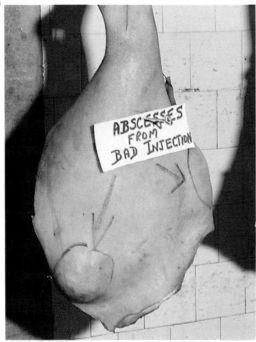

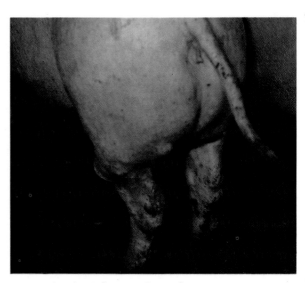

141 Injection abscess Granulomatous response in the left ham due to reaction after use of a vaccine with an unnamed oil emulsion adjuvant.

140 Injection abscesses in the ham of a 90 kg pig, caused through the use of a contaminated needle.

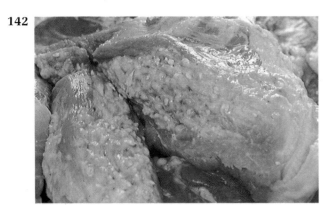

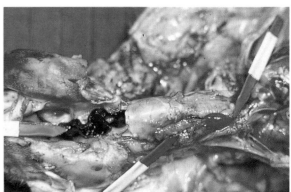

142 Injection abscess Cross-section of the granulomatous reaction featured in **141**.

143 Traumatic injury to the oesophagus resulting in perforation, possibly due to the faulty use of a dosing gun.

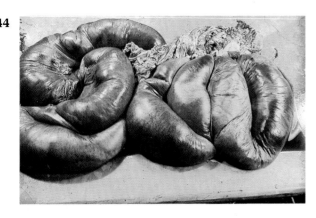

144 Unattended dystocia (gangrenous metritis) Uterus from a sow which was seen to have dystocia and was then left for 12 hours after first manual interference before veterinary attendance. The sow died an hour later with clostridial gangrene of the uterus.

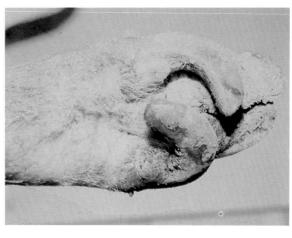

145 Overgrown supernumerary claws of a five-year-old sow housed on smooth concrete.

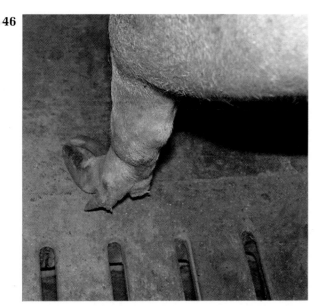

146 Overgrown claws Sow in part-slatted stall.

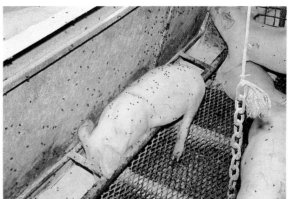

147 Fly infestation Fly problem in a weaner pen with underfloor slurry storage.

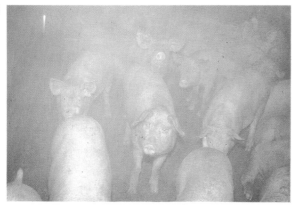

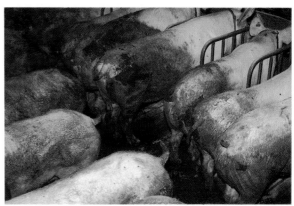

14

148 Excessive humidity This is not acceptable from a welfare point of view.

149 Perineal contamination Sows in tethered, slatted accommodation. Note the heavy contamination of the perineal area due to the slurry level rising above the slats – a situation predisposing to cystitis, vaginitis and infertility.

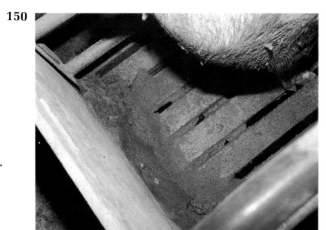

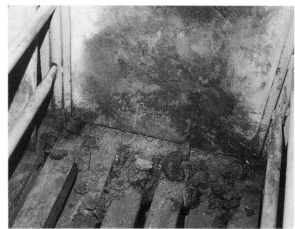

15

150 Perineal contamination A sow in a slatted stall, demonstrating how continual contamination of the perineal area occurs, predisposing to cystitis. This is due to the back gate extending to the floor (*see also* **151**).

151 Perineal contamination Note the build-up of faeces on the slats due to a back gate extending to the floor. Solid back gates should stop 10ʰm or so from the floor.

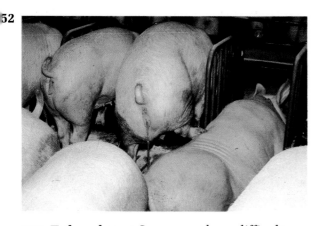

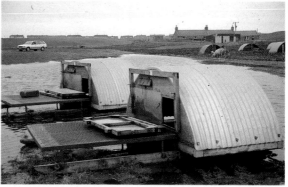

152 Tethered sows Some sows have difficulty in achieving the correct posture for micturition. This leads to urine retention – a predisposing factor in the development of cystitis.

153 Weaner units These weaner units were placed in a field and were successful for two years until extremes of weather brought a halt to their use.

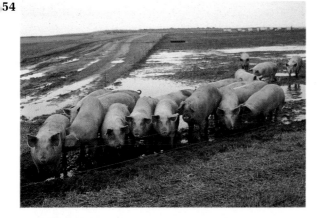

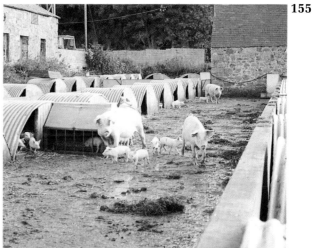

154 Dry sows In order to satisfy all welfare requirements these sows were given the freedom of a large grass field. However, weather extremes soon made the conditions unacceptable.

155 Farrowing arks Because of hostile weather conditions in winter, the farmer brought the arks into the shelter of the farm yard. This created conditions likely to cause disease – especially enteric disease.

156

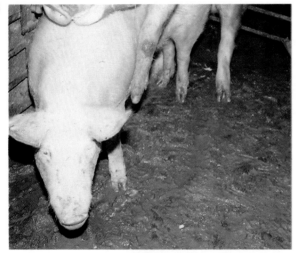

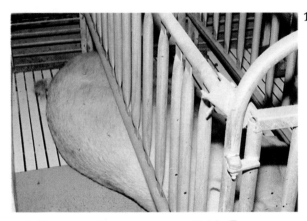

156 Boar serving sow on unsuitable floor
This is likely to lead to slipping and injury to
both.

157 Farrowing crate A sow in a farrowing
crate with the lower horizontal bar too far from
the floor, allowing the sow to become trapped,
leading to subsequent struggling and possible
injury to the back or spine. It should be noted
that the sow may be able to struggle free after
the injury has occurred.

158

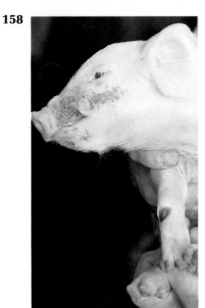

158 Facial necrosis in a 12-day-old piglet. A
result of bad tooth clipping technique.

159 Facial necrosis in five-day-old piglet due
to fighting with litter mates whose canine teeth
had not been clipped.

160 Multiple micro-abscesses on the udder
due to piercing of the skin by the unclipped
canine teeth of the piglets (*see* **435**).

159

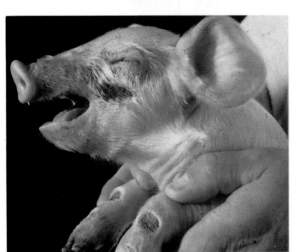

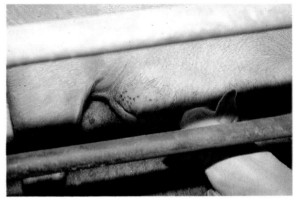

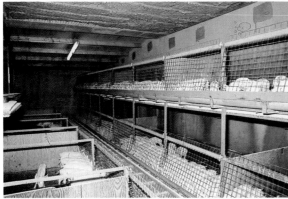

161 Tiered flat-deck accommodation Now considered unacceptable in the UK on welfare grounds. The piglets in this particular environmentally controlled weaner house performed well and did not appear to suffer from any welfare-related problems.

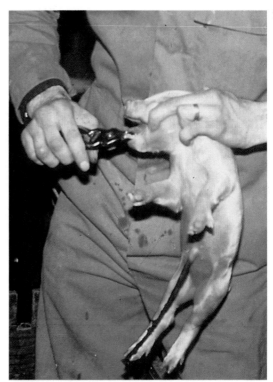

162 Clipping the canine (needle) teeth of a newborn piglet – a measure to prevent injury to the faces of littermates and to the udder of the sow.

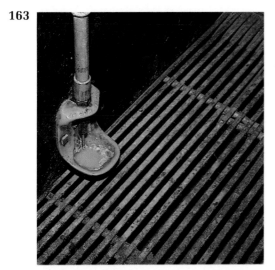

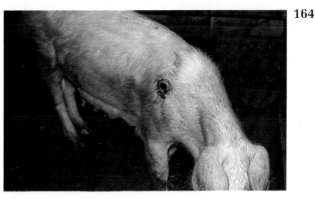

164 Sow with shoulder sore These are seen mainly over the spine of the scapula in modern hybrid sows during the suckling period. Severely affected sows are usually thin and should be housed on deep bedding.

163 Drinking bowl, heavily contaminated with piglet faeces. Piglets drinking from this bowl are liable to suffer from enteric problems.

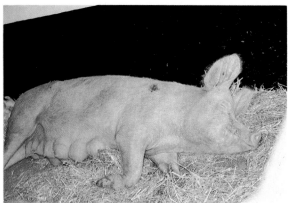

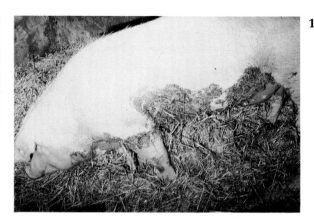

165 Sow with shoulder sore Although this sow was housed on straw bedding, pressure sores appeared because the bedding was not deep enough. A reduction in subcutaneous fat may have been a precipitating factor.

166 Burning Sow involved in a straw fire. Note the typical ventral distribution of the burn lesions and the sparing of the nipples which are cooled by secretions.

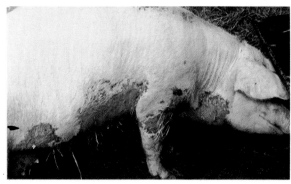

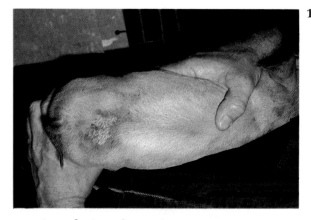

167 Burning Sow involved in a straw fire. The severe burn wounds seen here were colonised by bacteria such as *Bacillus cereus*.

168 Burn lesion This piglet had been burnt by an infra-red lamp which had been hung too low.

Disorders Relating to Trauma

The pig is in contact with the physical environment for almost all of its life. In practice this means that the skin of the abdomen, legs or claws will commonly be in apposition to the floor. In the natural situation the pigs' feet or claws are intended to be the hardware and the ground (floor) the software. Housing on concrete, or other man-made floors, has reversed this natural phenomenon, so that in intensive housing situations, the claws have become the software and the floor the hardware. This has resulted in a number of conditions, especially of the claws, becoming well-recognised. Abrasions with subsequent erosions often lead to septic laminitis, septic tenosynovitis, skin necrosis and adventitious bursitis.

169

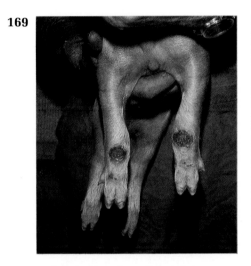

169 Knee necrosis in a five-day-old piglet.

170

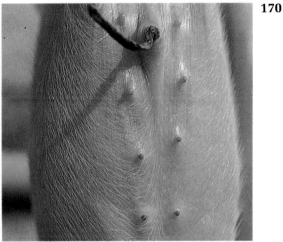

170 Nipple necrosis in a four-day-old piglet. Note that two anterior pairs of teats are affected.

171

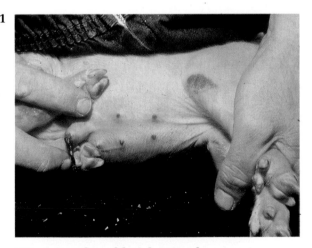

171 A two-day-old piglet Nipple necrosis, elbow necrosis, knee necrosis, hock necrosis and trauma with haemorrhage of feet at the sole/heel junction can be seen. All are due to contact with the floor.

172

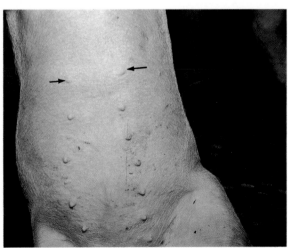

172 Weaner showing stunting of the anterior pair of teats (arrows) – a sequel to nipple necrosis.

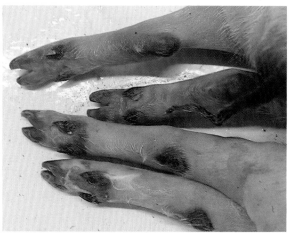

173 Tail necrosis and necrosis of the skin
overlying the hocks and accessory digits due to
abrasion on rough concrete.

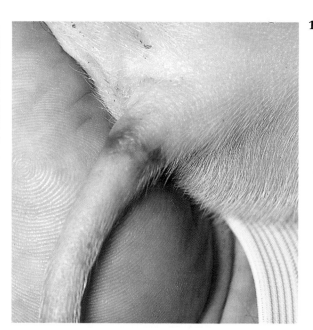

174 A two-day-old piglet Close-up of an early
lesion encircling the tail, produced by contact
with the floor. This will lead to tail necrosis.
Scalding from acute diarrhoea may also
produce such a lesion.

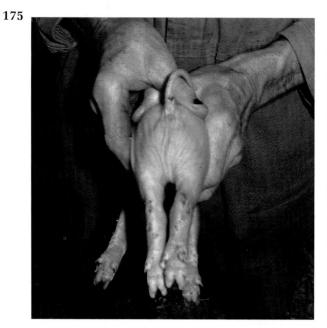

175 A two-day-old piglet Early traumatic
lesion on the underside of the tail. Constriction
of the scar, if it encircles the tail, will lead to
tail necrosis.

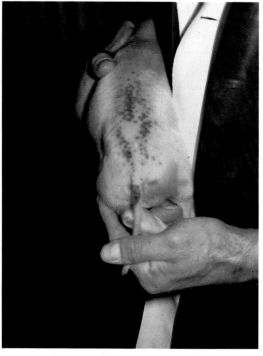

176 A three-day-old piglet Early traumatic
lesion with scarring on the tail head.

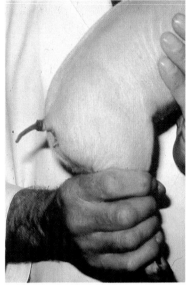

177 Tail necrosis in a five-day-old piglet.

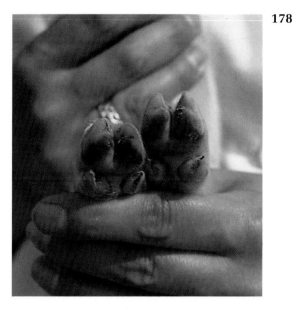

178 A two-day-old piglet on rough concrete
Note the severe bruising of the sole in all claws.

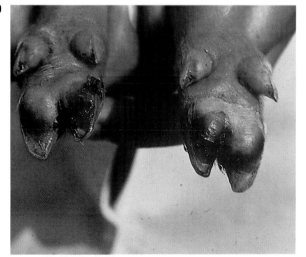

179 Erosion of the soles of mesial digits of the hind legs with haemorrhage. A three-day-old piglet on expanded metal.

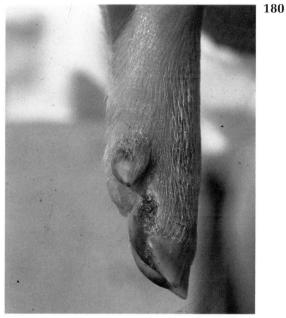

180 A five-day-old piglet on expanded metal
Note the damage to the heel bulb.

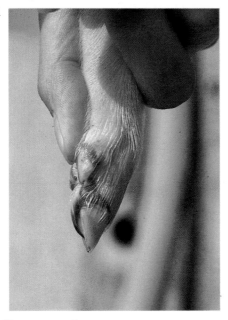

181 Damage to the coronary band of both supernumerary and main digits.

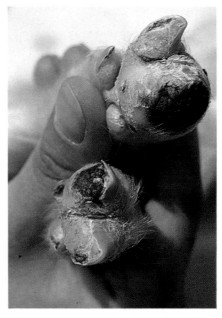

182 A 19-day-old piglet on expanded metal
Note the healing erosions of both soles (left foot) and chronic septic laminitis of the mesial claw (right foot).

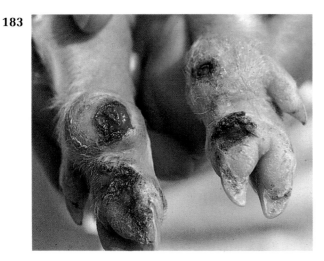

183 Chronic active erosions on both heel bulbs and severe damage to both mesial supernumerary digits.

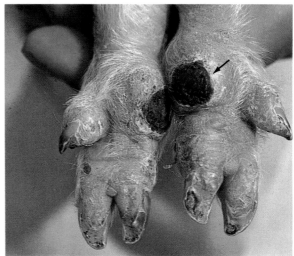

184 An 18-day-old piglet on expanded metal
Note the severe damage to the mesial supernumerary digits and healing erosions on the soles (arrows).

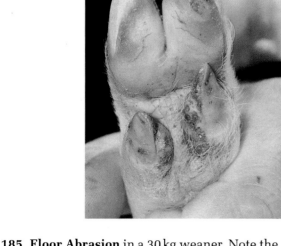

185 **Floor Abrasion** in a 30 kg weaner. Note the erosion of the sole (arrow).

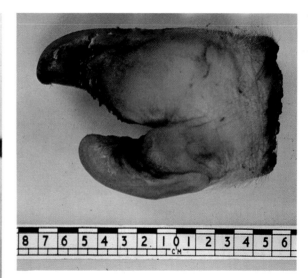

186 **Markedly unequal digits** (lateral larger) and early sole erosion.

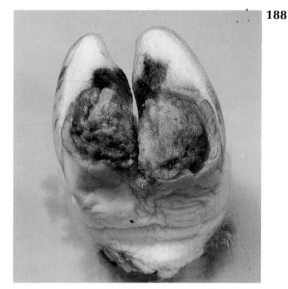

187 **Toe erosion** Lateral claw of a 60 kg pig. Note the difference in shape of the claws.

188 **Heel, sole and toe erosion** in the left hind foot of an 80 kg pig. Note the difference in shape of the claws.

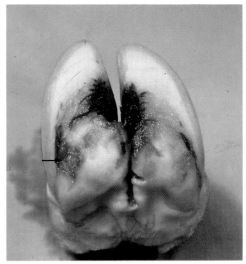

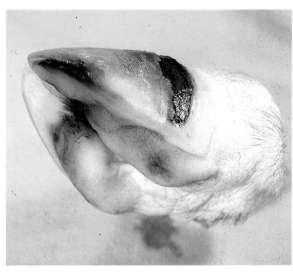

189 Toe erosions of both claws Right hind foot of a 60 kg pig. Note the early heel erosion (arrow).

190 White line lesion with penetration of the claw and separation at the coronary band in an 80 kg pig.

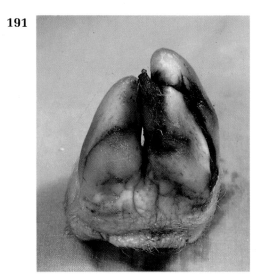

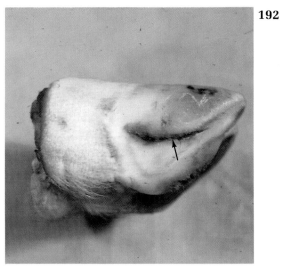

191 Severe white line lesion extending across the sole with some heel erosions and 'corn' formation. Note the unequal digit size and difference in shape of the digits. The left hind foot of an 80 kg pig.

192 False sand crack (arrow) in the right hind foot of an 80 kg pig. Early heel lesions can just be seen.

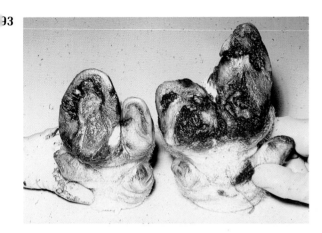

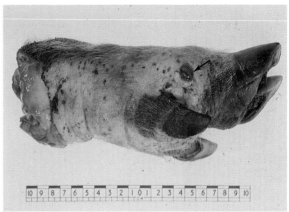

193 Feet of a Large-White boar culled because of severe lameness and inability to serve. Three claws developed bush-foot and there is severe heel erosion and ulceration.

194 Bush Foot in the right hind foot of a sow with a sinus above the claw (arrow). Note swelling.

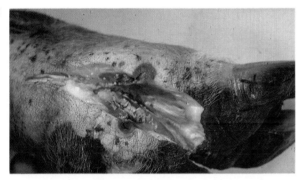

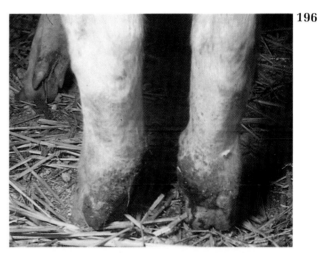

195 Bush Foot Right hind foot of the sow in **194**. The sinus above the claw has been incised to show a fibrino-necrotic lesion as a result of claw penetration and ascending infection.

196 Loss of supernumerary digits in a 28 kg weaner. Outbreaks have occurred and the digit loss is usually bilateral on the mesial aspect. The pig had been reared in a farrowing pen with a floor made of expanded metal (*see* **184**).

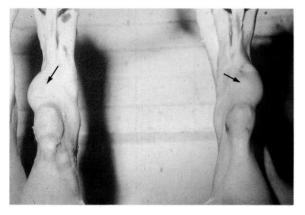

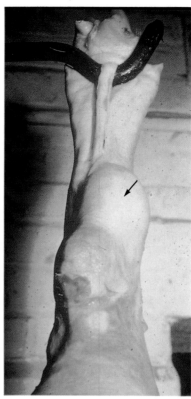

197 and **198 Adventitious bursitis of the hock**
(arrows) in 85 kg pigs at slaughter.

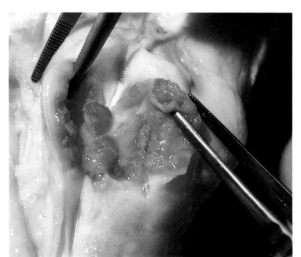

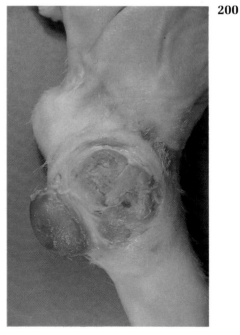

199 Bursa of the pig in **198**, incised showing
nodular hyperplasia of a false synovial
membrane.

**200 Advanced adventitious bursitis of the
hock** Note erosion of the dermis and most of
the bursal tissues, exposing the underlying
flesh. An 82 kg pig at slaughter.

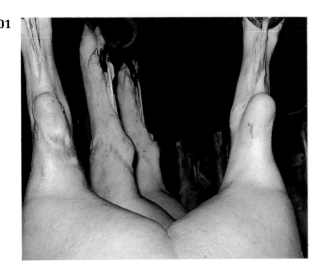

201 Bilateral bursitis (capped hock) in a 90 kg pig at slaughter.

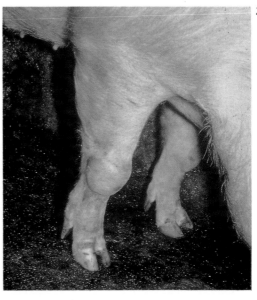

202 Bilateral carpal bursitis in a two-year-old sow.

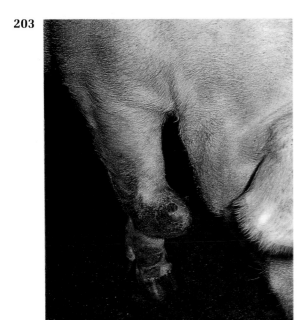

203 Carpal bursitis in a finishing pig. This lesion may be precipitated by difficulty in standing up.

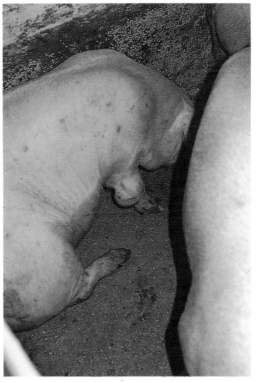

204 Capped elbow due to trauma in a finishing pig.

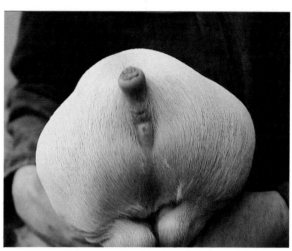

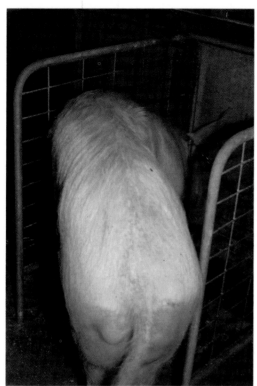

205 Bilateral bursae over tuber ischii.

206 Partial stenosis of the vulva A sequel to vulval necrosis. This is the piglet in **207** at 20 days of age.

207 Necrosis of the vulva A sequel to congenital oedema of the vulva with possible trauma (*see* **62**).

Parasitic Diseases

The common intestinal worms and lungworms are referred to as endoparasites. They are most likely to cause a problem in pigs reared in dirt lots, permanent pasture and strawed yards. Control can be achieved by a combination of clean pasture management and regular treatment with anthelmintics. Mange and lice infestation are the main ectoparasites. They have been eradicated from many herds and are easily controlled with the use of modern drugs.

Few parasites cause overt clinical disease in modern systems (with the exception of coccidia and mange) but most reduce productivity, and the photographs given here provide a guide to the parasites and the lesions by which they may be recognised.

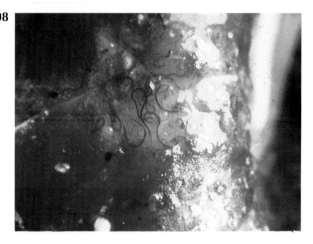

208 *Hyostrongylus rubidus* (Stomach worm) Heavy infestation may cause anaemia.

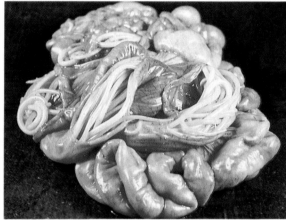

209 *Ascaris suum* Heavy infestation of adults in the small intestine.

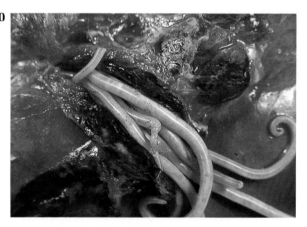

210 *Ascaris suum* Heavy infestation of the bile duct.

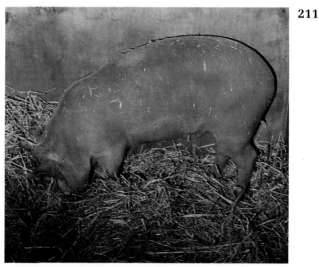

211 *Ascaris suum* Jaundiced, hypothermic 70 kg pig with *Ascaris* impaction in the bile duct.

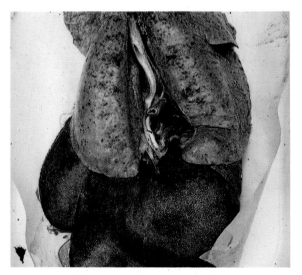

212 Ascaris suum Liver and lung from an 80 kg slaughter pig. Note the 'milk spot' liver and haemorrhages in the lung associated with more recent migration of larvae.

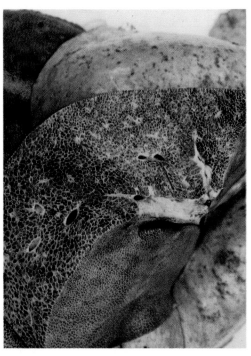

213 Ascaris suum Cut surface of the liver from **212** showing severe fibrosis throughout the liver.

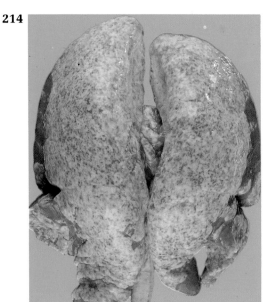

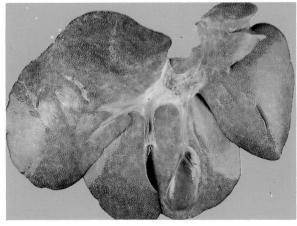

215 Ascaris suum Liver from the same experimental pig as in **214** (7 days post-infection) showing the lesions caused by migrating larvae.

214 Ascaris suum Lungs from one of four experimentally infected pigs showing the multiple petechial haemorrhages resulting from larval migration. Some peripheral collapse has also occurred.

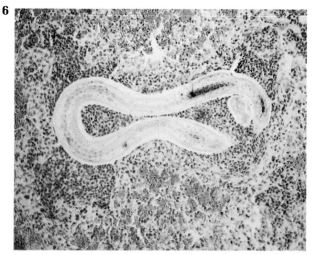

216 *Ascaris suum* Histological section showing a larva in the liver.

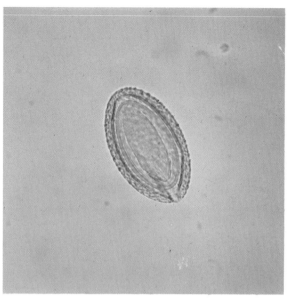

217 *Macracanthorhynchus hirudinaceus* Egg.

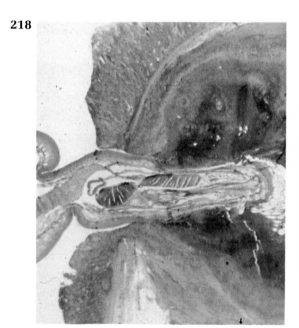

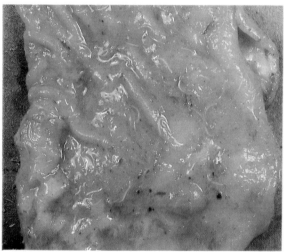

219 *Trichuris suis* Caecum from a 140 kg gilt with heavy infestation of *Trichuris suis*. Note the mucoid caecal contents.

218 *Macracanthorhynchus hirudinaceus* (Thorny-headed worm) Section through a head attached to the intestine.

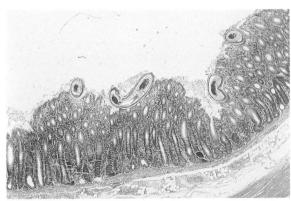

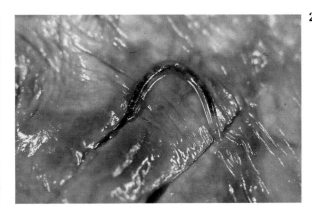

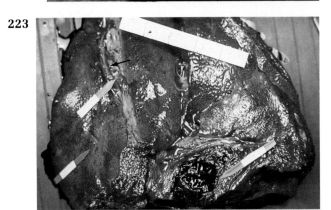

220 *Trichuris suis* Cross section of the caecum from **219** showing chronic active typhilitis. Several *Trichuris* worms can be seen in cross section.

221 *Stephanurus dentatus* **(Kidney worm)** This worm can also cause lesions in the liver, mesenteric lymph glands and other organs. The photograph shows a migrating worm in lung tissue.

222 *Metastrongylus apri* Note parasites in the bronchioles (arrow) and associated pneumonic lesions.

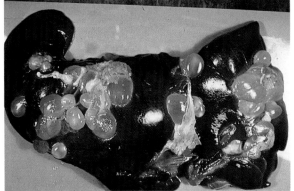

223 *Fasciola hepatica* Note flukes in the opened bile duct (arrow).

224 *Cysticercus tenuicollis* Cysts of *Taenia hydatigena* – a tapeworm of dogs and wild carnivores.

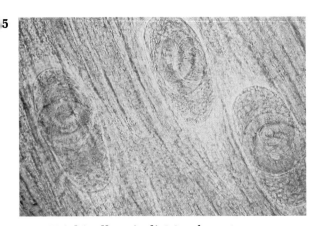

225 *Trichinella spiralis* Muscle cysts.

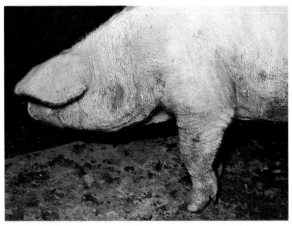

226 Sarcoptic mange in an 18-month-old gilt with severe mange due to infestation with *Sarcoptes scabei* var *suis*.

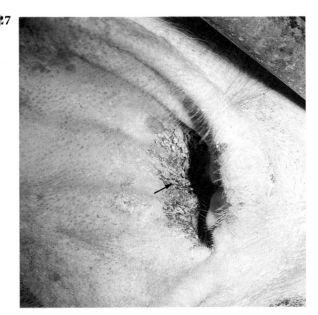

227 Chronic sarcoptic mange in a 3-year-old sow. Note the scab (arrow) at the base of the ear. The crumbly wax from such lesions is rich in mites (*see* **229**) and forms the most readily available source of material for the confirmation of diagnosis.

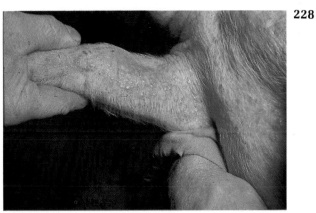

228 Sarcoptic mange Weaner pig with typical skin lesions indicative of hypersensitivity to the presence of mange mites.

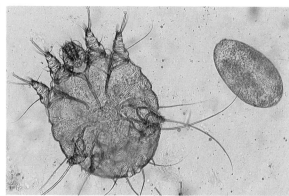

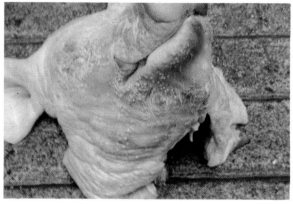

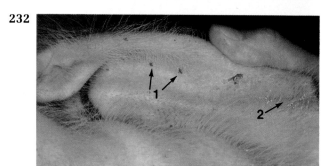

231

229 Sarcoptic mange *Sarcoptes* mite (adult female) and egg.

230 Demodectic mange (*Demodex folliculorum* var *suis*) Rarely seen clinically, the pustules present on the lips and jowl of this slaughter pig were teeming with the typical fusiform mites.

231 Demodectic mange Nodular lesions on the skin of a bacon pig. These develop into pustules which often contain Staphylococci.

232

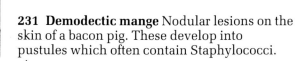

232 Lice (*Haematopinus suis*) Lice may be found over the whole body but at times may retreat to extremities such as the feet. They are often to be found inside the pinna of the ear (1) and on hairs here and on the neck, the nits or eggs can be seen (2). Between the two sets of arrows is a louse feeding site.

233

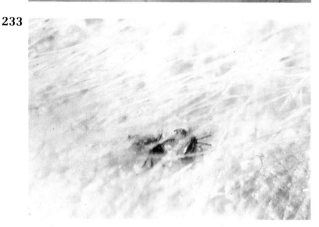

233 Lice Close-up of adult lice feeding.

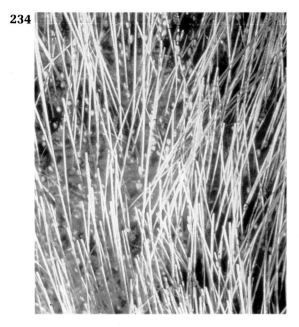

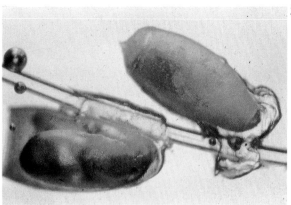

235 Lice Close-up of eggs deposited on hair.

234 Lice Close-up of severe egg (nit) infestation.

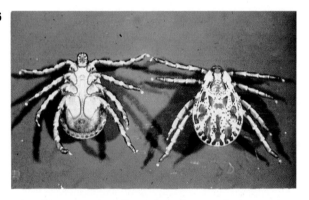

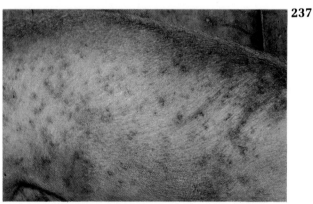

236 *Dermacentor* Dorsal and ventral views of male ticks. Ticks may spread viral diseases such as louping ill and swine pox. Swine pox can also be spread by lice.

237 Biting lesions Skin lesions associated with mosquito or fly bites.

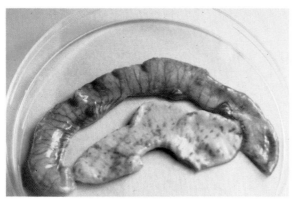

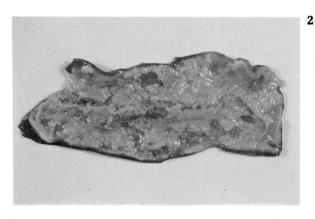

238 Coccidiosis (*Isospora suis*) Ileum from a 10-day-old piglet thickened by coccidiosis. Note the opaque serosal surface and the thickened wall. The contents contain necrotic material.

239 Coccidiosis (*Isospora suis*) Small intestine of an 8-day-old piglet. Note necrosis of the mucosa.

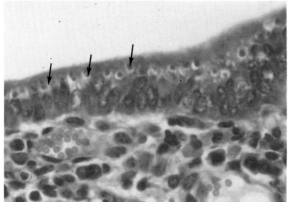

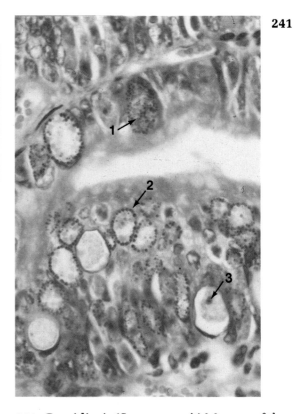

240 Coccidiosis (*Isospora suis*) Small intestine mucosa showing undifferentiated parasites (often binucleate) which appear to occupy every host cell (arrows).

241 Coccidiosis (*Isospora suis*) Mucosa of the small intestine showing infection of enterocytes with coccidia in various stages of maturation including microgamonts (1), macrogamonts (2), and young oocysts (3).

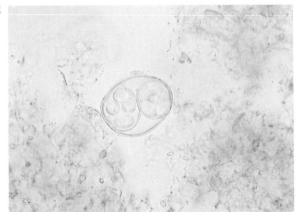

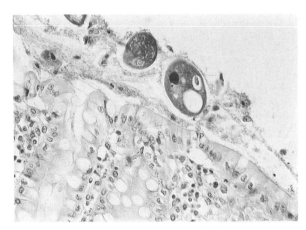

242 Coccidiosis (*Isospora suis*) Sporulated oocyst.

243 *Balantidium coli* is present in low numbers in the large intestines of normal pigs but increases in numbers dramatically when gut function is disturbed. Its role in disease is not yet clear but it may be seen on the lumenal surface of the large intestinal mucosa in histological sections or in wet smears of fresh tissue. Cysts or even active organisms may be seen in fresh smears of diarrhoeic faeces.

Fungal Diseases

Fungi may cause a variety of diseases which may be due directly to fungal invasion of tissue (such as ringworm) or more often to the ingestion of toxins produced by fungi in growing, standing or stored grains and other feeds. Several of these toxins may produce no gross lesions, but may be evident at histopathological level. Several may, however, produce specific clinical signs but these are not common.

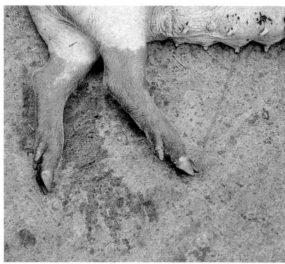

244 Ergot poisoning Sow showing bilateral hind limb lesions. Ergot (*Claviceps purpurea*) may be ingested from contaminated grain containing sclerotia or on grass from infested pastures in late summer and autumn. Abortion may result and necrosis of the extremities may be seen in severe cases. However, the pig is considered *very resistant* to ergot poisoning, although a form of agalactia has been reported.

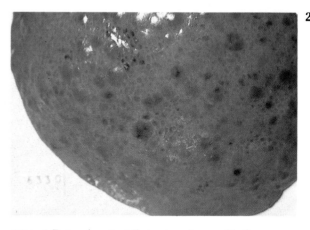

245 Aflatoxicosis Aflatoxicosis results from the ingestion of ready-formed Aflatoxin from protein or maize-based concentrates in which *Aspergillus flavus* has multiplied. As this toxin is highly carcinogenic, this material is controlled under the Aflatoxicosis Order, 1980.

The liver shown here is tan in colour with a nodular surface due to the widespread necrosis and damage caused by ingested toxin. Haemorrhages and jaundice may be present in the carcase.

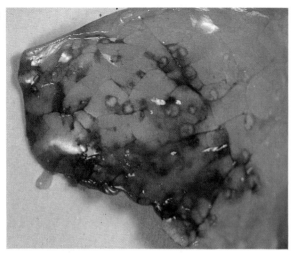

246 *Aspergillus flavus* Lung lesions. Systemic infection with this fungus is rare.

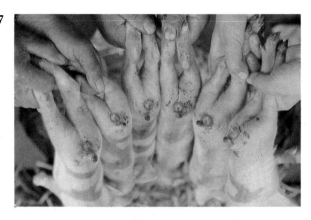

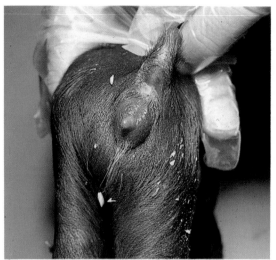

247–249 Fusariotoxicosis Congenital oedema of the vulva in piglets born to dams with 'mouldy corn poisoning' resulting from high levels of Zearalenone (F–2 toxin) in the dam (*see also* **62**).

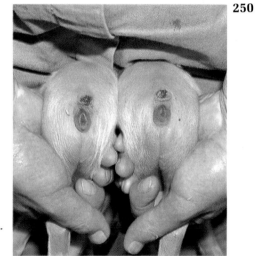

250 Vulval swelling in piglets of uncertain aetiology. Suspected fusariotoxicosis. *Single* cases like this within a litter are quite common in the UK.

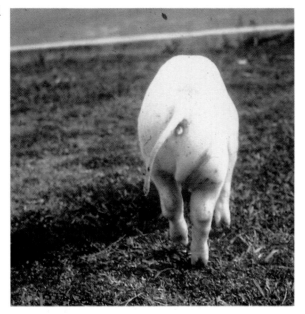

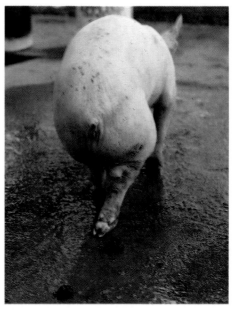

251 Mycotoxicosis Haematoma at an injection site in a case of mycotoxicosis due to eating mouldy bread. Note blood-staining of the anal area. (Tricothecene toxins were suspected and the animals responded to synthetic vitamin K in feed).

252 Mycotoxicosis Haemarthrosis of right stifle joint due to mouldy corn poisoning. The same outbreak as **251**.

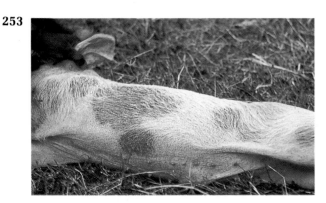

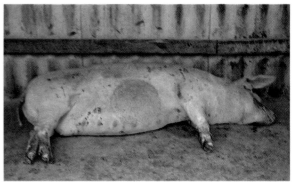

253 Ringworm Weaner with skin lesions due to *Microsporum nanum*. Not reported in the UK, this ringworm fungus is the most common species affecting the pig worldwide. Little irritation is associated with ringworm infection in pigs.

254 Ringworm *Microsporum nanum* infection in a gilt at the point of farrowing.

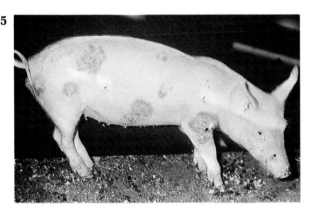

255 *Microsporum nanum* infection in a grower.

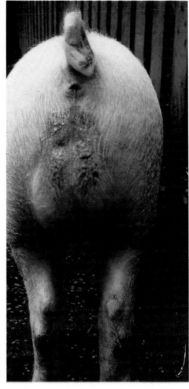

256 Ringworm Boar with scrotal lesions due to *Trichophyton mentagrophytes.*

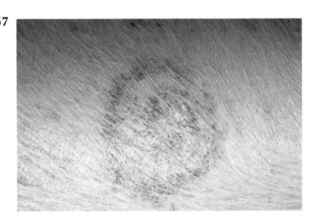

257 *Trichophyton verrucosum* infection.

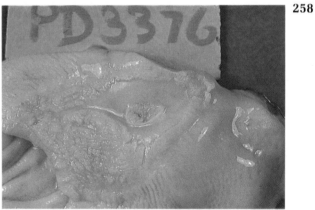

258 *Candida albicans* infection of the stomach. Note the plaque-like lesions in the pars oesophagea. *Candida* infections are commonly associated with depressed immunity or imbalance of the gut flora after continuous intake of antibiotic.

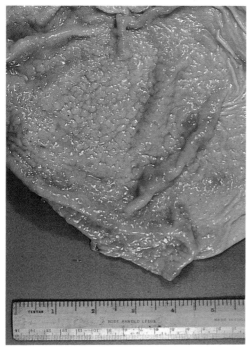

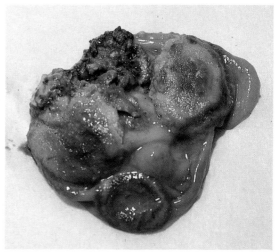

260 Mucormycosis Stomach from a seven-day-old piglet with lesions of mucormycosis due to dam receiving high levels of chlortetracycline in feed.

259 Mucormycosis Stomach showing raised circular lesions. *Mucor* is not a primary pathogen for the pig intestine and usually colonises existing lesions of immunosuppressed pigs.

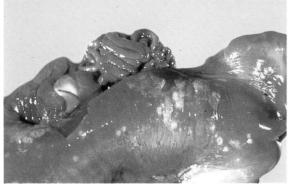

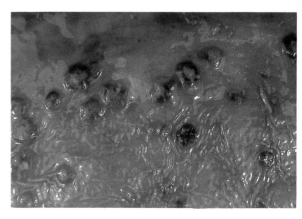

261 Mycotic Abortion Note the skin lesions on the foetus. These contain actively growing colonies of the fungus. (Species not identified).

262 Mycotic Abortion Placental lesions (species not identified).

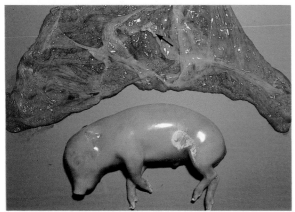

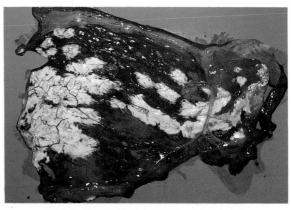

263 Fungal abortion due to *Aspergillus* infection. Note the plaques on both the piglet and placenta (arrow).

264 Placental plaques. A *normal* finding on many placentae.

Bacterial Diseases

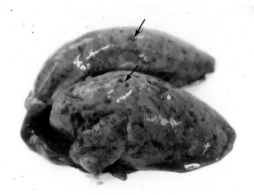

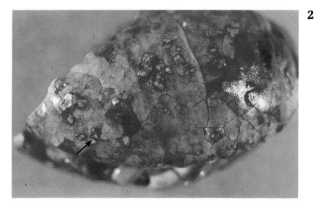

266 *Actinobacillus suis* Lungs from a five-day-old piglet. Note the miliary abscesses (arrow), the oedema and the congestion.

265 Actinobacillosis *Actinobacillus suis* causes septicaemia in neonates, vegetative endocarditis, arthritis in slightly older pigs and pleuropneumonia in older animals. These lungs are from a case of neonatal septicaemia and show the most obvious lesions (arrows). Histological lesions are pathognomonic and consist of areas of necrosis containing microcolonies of the organism.

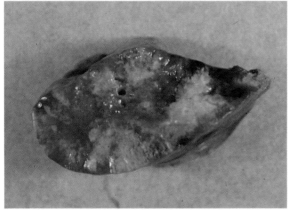

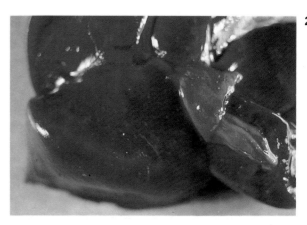

267 *Actinobacillus suis* Section through the lung shown in **266**. Note the mottled appearance and the areas of pneumonia.

268 *Actinobacillus suis* Liver from a case of *A. suis* septicaemia in a five-day-old piglet. Pinhead yellowish microabscesses can be seen on the surface of the liver.

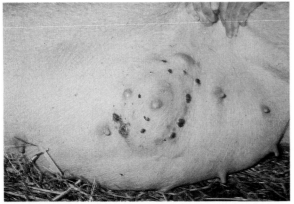

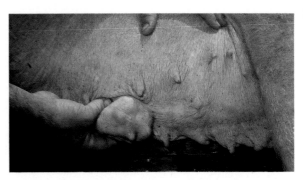

269 Actinobacillosis *Actinobacillus lignieresi* infection of the udder of a sow. Note the hard lumps made prominent by stretching the skin and the multiple scabs around the nipple. These represent temporarily-healed sinuses where the underlying granulomas have discharged to the exterior.

270 Actinobacillosis Hard, granulomatous lesions in one or more mammae of the sow's udder are often described as 'Actinobacillosis'. In some cases, actinobacilli can be isolated and the diagnosis confirmed; in others, staphylococci are isolated. Note the firm nature of the lesions in the udder.

Bacillus anthracis (Anthrax)

Anthrax may occur as a septicaemia in which case pigs are found dead, or as a localised infection of the submandibular lymph nodes or small intestine.

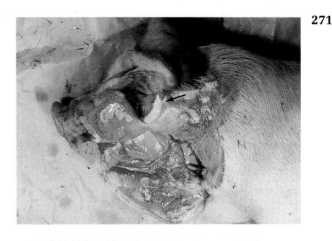

271

271 Anthrax A pig which has recently died from anthrax. Note the thickened and oedematous skin (arrow) and the enlarged lymph nodes. Smears made from this area often contain the bacilli which are often not visible in conventional blood smears.

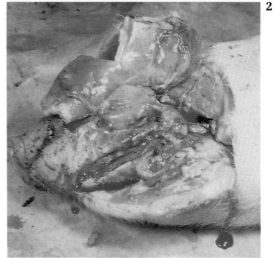

272

272 Anthrax A pig which has died of anthrax. Note the swollen jowl and the fluid running from the wound.

Brucella suis and infertility

B. suis infects both sows and boars, causing infertility. Infection in sows can cause returns to oestrus five to eight weeks after service and infection later in pregnancy gives rise to mummified, stillborn or weak pigs. Copious blood-stained vulval discharge and endo-metritis occur. In boars testicular swelling, orchitis and epididymitis may develop within seven weeks of infection and the testicles may atrophy later in the disease. Osteomyelitis and arthritis may also be seen.

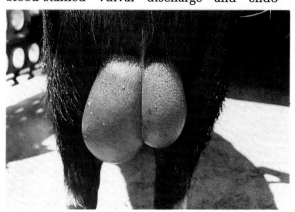

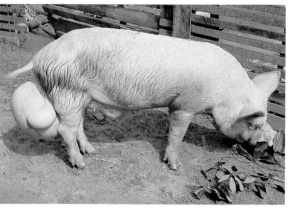

27

273 *Brucella suis* This boar has enlargement of the left testicle caused by infection with *B. suis*.

274 *Brucella suis* A large white boar with *B. suis* orchitis. Note the enlargement of the testis.

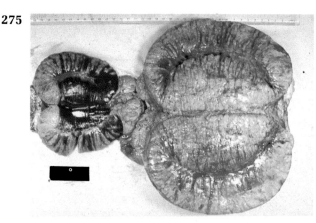

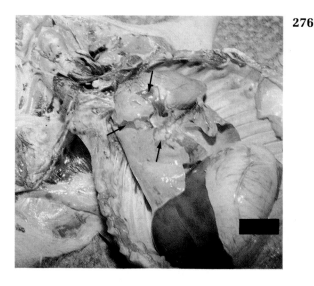

275 *Brucella suis* Longitudinal section of porcine testes illustrating degrees of orchitis due to *B. suis* infection. The gross enlargement of the testis on the right is due to necrosis of the seminiferous tubules with thickening of the interstitial tissue. The smaller testicle on the left contains pale areas of necrotic seminiferous tubules.

276 *Bordetella bronchiseptica* The most common lesions of *Bordetella* pneumonia are those of lobular collapse, seen here as incidental findings in a four-week-old pig from a flat deck weaner unit. Note the distribution of the lesions (arrows).

277 ***Bordetella bronchiseptica*** causes rhinitis and bronchitis in young non-immune pigs. When the bronchitis is severe, mucus and pus accumulate in the bronchioles and may be inspired to cause pneumonia. This may be fatal, or it may depress growth. Early lesions are shown in this photograph. The organism can be isolated from both bronchi and lesions at this stage.

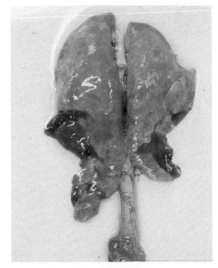

277

278 ***Bordetella bronchiseptica*** The distal portion of a cranial lung lobe showing lesions typical of *Bordetella bronchiseptica* pneumonia and its consequences. The dark areas of collapse surround pale areas of over-inflation.

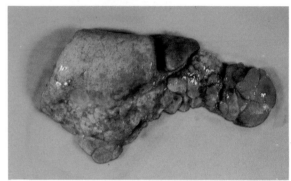

278

Clostridium perfringens type C enteritis

Clostridium perfringens type C causes a severe enteritis in neonatal pigs characterised by the passage of bloodstained diarrhoea, and death in those less than four days old. Slightly older pigs may survive but are often stunted due to necrotic enteritis. The clinical signs and the post mortem findings are usually sufficient for a diagnosis to be made. The disease is confirmed by demonstration of the organism and its toxin in gut contents.

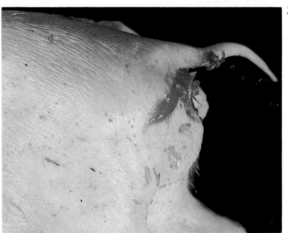

279

279 ***Clostridium perfringens*** **type C enteritis** The bloodstained faeces shown here is typical of that seen in affected neonatal pigs.

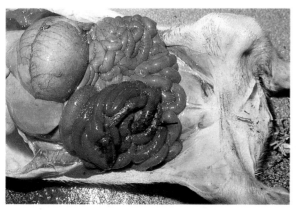

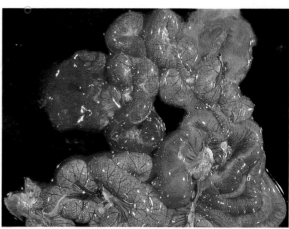

28

280 *Clostridium perfringens* **type C enteritis**
Close-up of the haemorrhagic intestines of a
piglet which has died from this disease. Note
the heavily-congested areas where roughening
of the intestinal wall has resulted from a
combination of gas formation in the wall and
intense local peritonitis (arrow).

281 *Clostridium perfringens* **type C enteritis**
Small intestine of a neonatal piglet with
Clostridium perfringens type C enteritis
opened to demonstrate the bloodstained nature
of the contents.

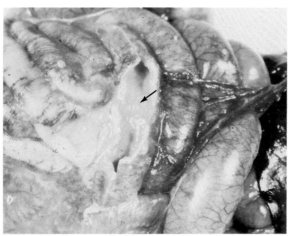

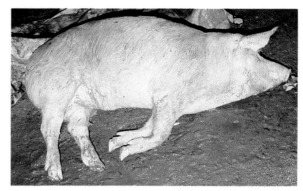

283 *Clostridium novyi* (*oedematiens*) Large
finishing pigs or sows may die suddenly as a
result of infection with *Clostridium novyi*.
Animals are usually in good condition and
markedly bloated. This photograph shows the
carcase of one such pig which was one of seven
heavy hogs to die on a swill-fed unit over a
period of one month.

282 *Clostridium perfringens* **type C enteritis**
Small intestine from a chronic case. Note
necrosis and thickening of the bowel wall
(arrow).

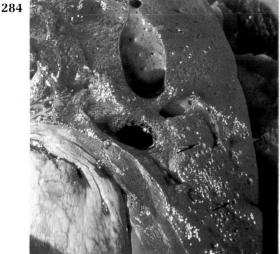

284 Clostridium novyi (oedematiens) The livers of pigs which have died from *Clostridium novyi* infection contain cavities similar to those shown here (arrow). Similar cavities also develop during post mortem decomposition, and diagnosis depends on the demonstration of the organism in the lesions, the freshness of the carcase and the success of vaccination in prevention.

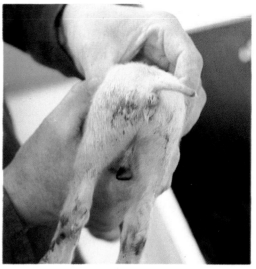

285 Clostridium perfringens type A enteritis This condition occurs in neonatal piglets and is rarely fatal. Pasty, mucoid diarrhoea begins within 12–36 hours of birth and affected piglets lose condition and develop the perineal faecal staining shown here in this 48-hour-old piglet.

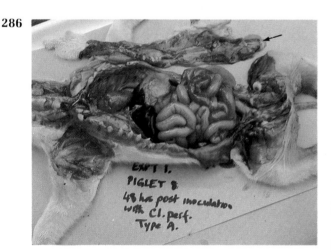

286 Clostridium perfringens type A enteritis Piglets which die from the disease often develop subnormal body temperatures prior to death and show marked blackening of the abdominal skin surface. This animal was killed in the terminal stages of the disease. Note the blackened abdominal skin (arrow), the congested carcase and the distended, gas-filled intestines.

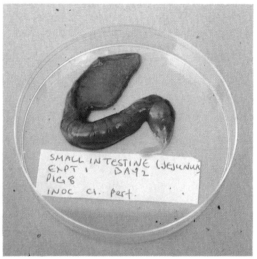

287 Clostridium perfringens type A enteritis Small intestine from a case of *Clostridium perfringens* type A infection in a neonatal piglet. The intestine is reddened and dilated with fluid, and the mucosa is covered with small patches of necrotic material.

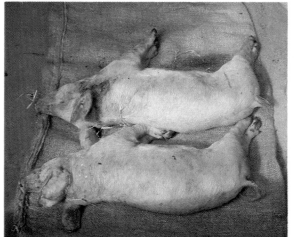

288 *Clostridium tetani* **(Tetanus)** Two live weaned pigs in tetanic spasm. Note the pricked ears and rigidly extended limbs. Infection had entered by way of contaminated castration wounds. Both pigs recovered.

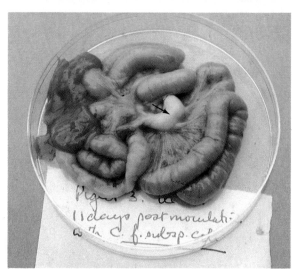

Campylobacter coli

Campylobacter coli infection occurs in most pigs soon after birth. Maternal immunity normally protects against any disease, but occasionally a new strain of organism can cause a mucoid diarrhoea. The organism also colonises any inflammatory lesion of the intestine as a secondary invader. When it is involved in enteritis, there is thickening of the small intestinal wall and enlargement of the mesenteric lymph nodes.

289 *Campylobacter coli* Thickened ileum of a piglet experimentally infected with *Campylobacter coli*. Note the enlarged lymph nodes (arrow) and pale, thickened ileal wall.

Porcine Proliferative Enteropathies

The porcine intestinal adenomatosis complex (known in the USA as the Ileitis Complex) comprises a number of conditions in which the underlying lesion is adenomatous proliferation of the mucosal epithelium. Porcine intestinal adenomatosis (PIA) is the primary condition. It is seen most commonly in the weaned pig (six to 12 weeks old) and is typified by anorexia and wasting. Diarrhoea is infrequent unless there is associated mucosal necrosis. Necrotic enteritis (NE) and regional ileitis (RI) occur in the same age group of pig as PIA. In these two conditions diarrhoea frequently occurs with anorexia and wasting. In NE there is massive necrosis of adenomatous mucosa. The main feature of RI is the rigidity of the affected bowel due to muscular hypertrophy and inflammatory change in the submucosa and lamina propria.

Proliferative haemorrhagic enteropathy (PHE) is more frequent in older pigs (16 weeks and upwards) and is characterised by an illness of shorter duration. Pigs are pale, may be seen passing tarry, black faeces, or may just be found dead. The main feature of PHE is the presence in the intestinal lumen of clotted blood, often in the form of a cast with clotted fibrin and necrotic tissue. The clots are commonly seen in the terminal ileum, the mucosa of which is thickened and adenomatous.

Histological lesions of intestinal adenomatosis are characteristic. There is thickening of the terminal ileal and/or large intestinal mucosa due to epithelial proliferation. This proliferation results in the development of long crypts lined with elongated epithelial cells. Campylobacter-like organisms can be demonstrated in the apical cytoplasm of the adenomatous epithelial cells by silver stains and immunofluorescence. Intracellular campylobacters can be identified in mucosal impression smears stained by Koster's differential staining method used to demonstrate brucellae.

A number of campylobacters have been recovered from adenomatous mucosa in affected pigs, but the organism which appears to be responsible has not yet been isolated in pure culture.

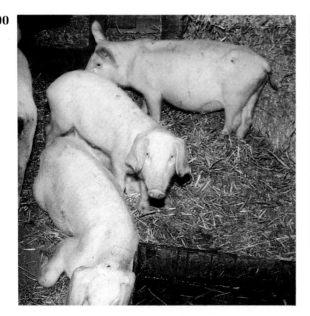

290 Proliferative Intestinal Adenomatosis (PIA) Affected 12-week-old pigs. Note their poor condition and pot bellies.

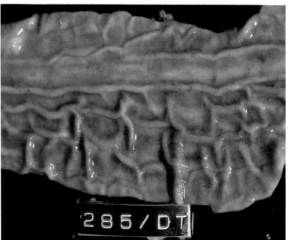

291 Proliferative Intestinal Adenomatosis Inflammation of the anterior ileal mucosa.

292

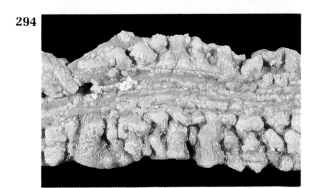

293

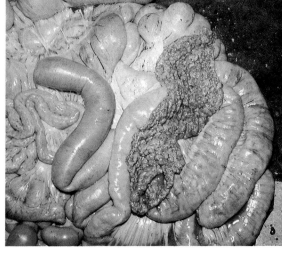

294

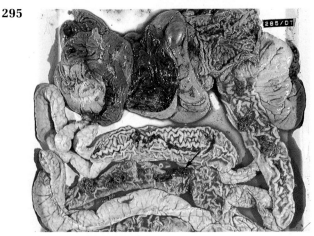

295

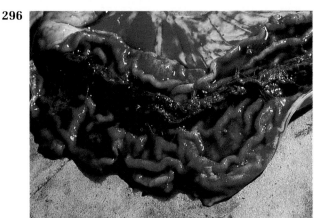

296

292 Regional ileitis (RI) At this late stage of the proliferative intestinal adenopathy process, the proliferated mucosa has almost filled the lumen of the gut on the left while muscular hypertrophy has caused rigidity of the bowel on the right. The bowel wall is weakened and may rupture; a generalised peritonitis results.

293 Necrotic enteritis (NE) Terminal ileum of a pig with necrotic enteritis. Note the distended bowel, through the wall of which pale patches can be seen. The opened portion shows the necrotic, formerly proliferative mucosa.

294 Necrotic enteritis (NE) Necrotic enteritis of the ileum in which the proliferative changes of PIA have become necrotic.

295 Proliferative Haemorrhagic Enteropathy (PHE) Intestinal tract from a case of proliferative haemorrhagic enteropathy. Note the presence of a blood clot in the ileum (arrow), the corrugated mucosa of the ileum and the reddened appearance of the large intestinal contents. This reddening is largely due to blood passing from the ileum.

296 Proliferative Haemorrhagic Enteropathy (PHE) Terminal ileum opened to show the blood clot in the lumen.

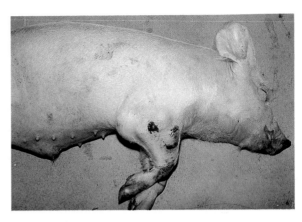

297 *Actinomyces (Corynebacterium) pyogenes* A. (C.) pyogenes is involved in abscesses in many different parts of the body. Here the left elbow joint of a 32 kg weaner is affected by septic arthritis and is enlarged.

298 *Actinomyces (C.) pyogenes* Carcase of a growing pig with gross lesions of septic arthritis from which *A. pyogenes* was isolated. Note the swollen right elbow.

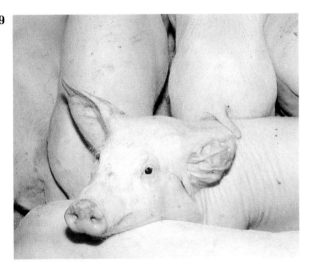

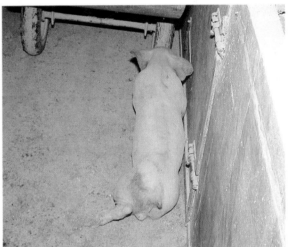

299 *Actinomyces (C.) pyogenes* A. (C.) *pyogenes* abscesses frequently occur in the spine, often as a result of tail biting (**654–660**). In this picture, a 24 kg weaner is seen in a position typical of paralysis, seated and immobile amongst a group of active pen-mates.

300 *Actinomyces (C.) pyogenes* The pig in **299**, shown on its own to demonstrate the extent of the paralysis.

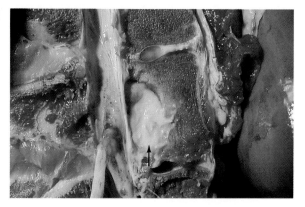

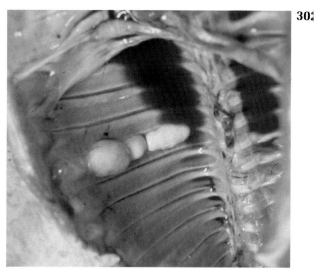

301 *Actinomyces (C.) pyogenes* Spinal abscess in the paralysed pig shown in **299**. Note the site of the abscess (arrow) in the vertebral body and the way it can compress the spinal cord to cause paralysis. In some cases the vertebral body collapses. The pus is typical of that produced in *A. (C.) pyogenes* infection; uniform in consistency; white, greyish-white or greenish-white in colour; and may smell foul.

302 *Actinomyces (C.) pyogenes* Abscesses on the parietal pleura along a rib. An incidental finding at post mortem examination of a weaner.

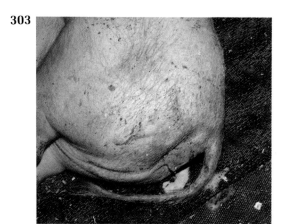

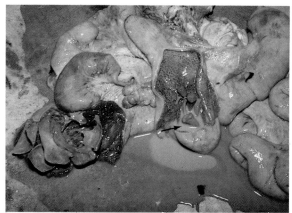

303 *Actinomyces (C.) pyogenes* Septic endometritis in a sow post-farrowing due to *A. (C.) pyogenes*. Note the vaginal discharge.

304 *Actinomyces (C.) pyogenes* Intra-uterine infection may result in complete digestion of the foetus to leave only the bones in a pool of pus (arrow). However, it may not be the original cause of death of the foetus.

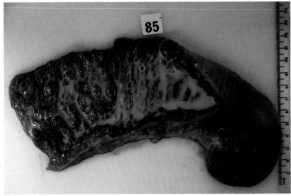

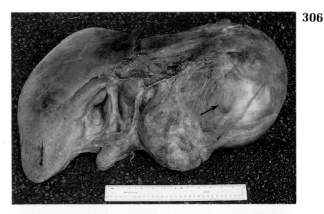

305 *Actinomyces (C.) pyogenes* Septic endometritis in sow uterus. Note the pus on the inflamed endometrium.

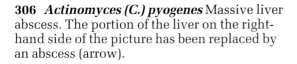

306 *Actinomyces (C.) pyogenes* Massive liver abscess. The portion of the liver on the right-hand side of the picture has been replaced by an abscess (arrow).

307 *Actinomyces (C.) pyogenes* Severe septic pericarditis which caused the death of a 35 kg pig. Note the creamy pus.

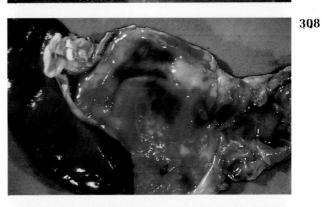

308 *Eubacterium (C.) suis* A congenitally-lobulated kidney with a massively enlarged and inflamed ureter caused by *E. suis* infection ascending from the bladder.

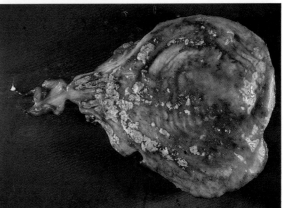

309 *Eubacterium (C.) suis* Bladder of a sow with acute cystitis due to infection with *E. suis*. Note the purulent material and the inflamed mucosa.

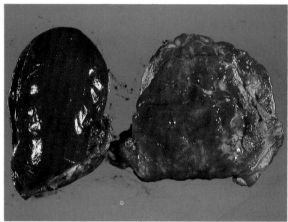

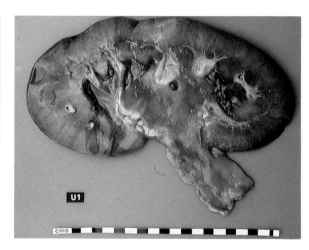

310 *Eubacterium (C.) suis* Kidney and bladder of a sow with *E. suis* infection. Note the inflamed mucosa of the bladder. In some cases there may be severe congestion of the kidney.

311 *Eubacterium (C.) suis* Longitudinal section of kidney from a sow with pyelonephritis caused by *E. suis* infection. Note the inflamed pelvis and the massively dilated ureter. Pus from the urine, bladder wall, ureter and kidney pelvis contains Gram-positive rods.

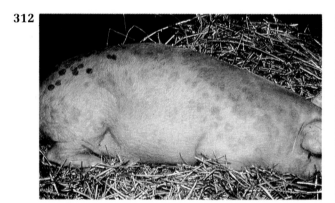

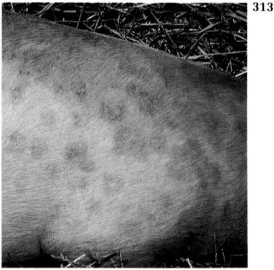

312 *Erysipelothrix rhusiopathiae* infection (Erysipelas) Pig with subacute erysipelas. The skin lesions are typical. On the hind leg the raised nature of the lesions can be clearly seen.

313 *Erysipelothrix rhusiopathiae* infection (Erysipelas) Closer view of the typical skin lesions of subacute erysipelas shown in **312**.

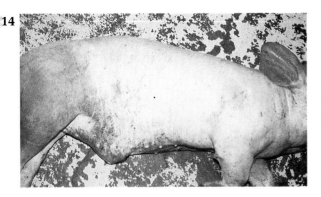

314 *Erysipelothrix rhusiopathiae* infection (Erysipelas) Chronic erysipelas may result from persisting infection in the heart valves to give a valvular endocarditis. Affected pigs of any age may show clinical signs of heart failure such as cyanosis of the extremities or be found dead. The carcase of this 30 kg pig, which died from vegetative endocarditis, shows this congestion over the hindquarters and on the ears.

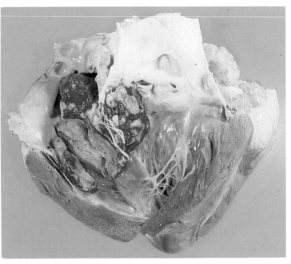

315 *Erysipelothrix rhusiopathiae* infection (Erysipelas) A heart from a pig with chronic erysipelas vegetative endocarditis. Note the large vegetations on the atrio-ventricular valves.

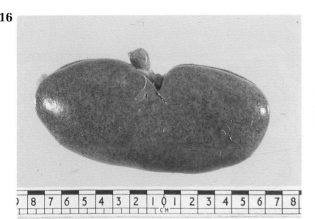

316 *Erysipelothrix rhusiopathiae* infection (Erysipelas) Kidney lesions in acute erysipelas. These are not common.

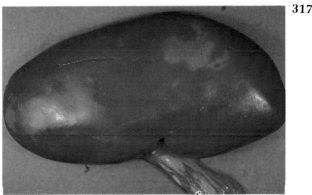

317 *Erysipelothrix rhusiopathiae* infection (Erysipelas) A kidney from a pig with vegetative endocarditis resulting from chronic erysipelas. Note the pale area of the infarct on the cortex of the kidney at top right.

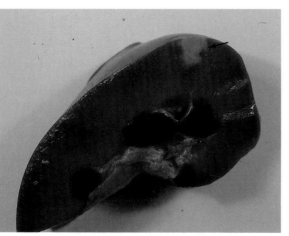

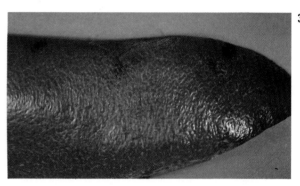

31

319 *Erysipelothrix rhusiopathiae* **infection (Erysipelas)** Spleen from a 70 kg pig which died with vegetative endocarditis caused by *E. rhusiopathiae*. Infarcts can be seen as dark patches.

318 *Erysipelothrix rhusiopathiae* **infection (Erysipelas)** A kidney from a pig with chronic erysipelas vegetative endocarditis, sectioned to show a pale infarct caused by an embolus (arrow).

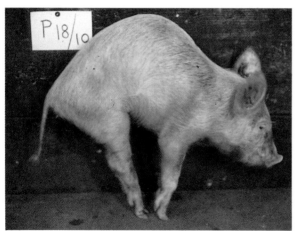

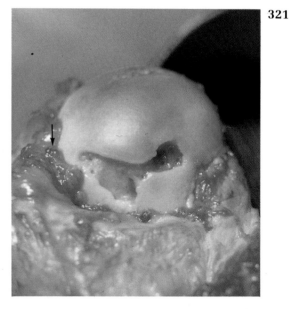

320 *Erysipelothrix rhusiopathiae* **infection (Erysipelas)** Weaner showing clinical signs of chronic erysipelas. The arthritis resulting from the localisation of the organism in the joints has produced a severe lameness.

321 *Erysipelothrix rhusiopathiae* **infection (Erysipelas)** Arthritis in chronic erysipelas from infection of the joint cavity and the subsequent proliferation of the synovial tissue. The femoral head shown here illustrates the hyperaemia and proliferation of the synovial membrane (arrow) and the erosion of the cartilage which occasionally accompanies it.

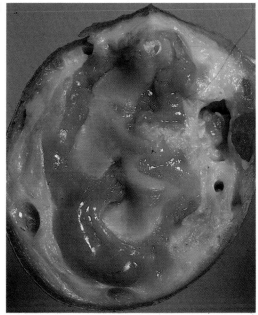

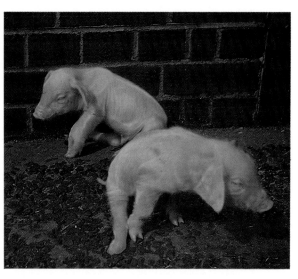

323 *Erysipelothrix rhusiopathiae* infection (Erysipelas) Congenital erysipelas in two newborn piglets. Note their inability to walk and the swollen joint of the far piglet. Erysipelas in pregnancy can cause abortion.

322 *Erysipelothrix rhusiopathiae* infection (Erysipelas) An arthritic joint with synovitis and pannus formation.

Glasser's Disease (*Haemophilus parasuis* infection)

Glasser's disease (*Haemophilus parasuis* infection) results in septicaemia, meningitis, arthritis, polyserositis and local lesions caused by clotting in blood vessels. Affected pigs may die in the acute stage of the disease, especially in non-immune herds, or from its chronic consequences. Weaner/growers are commonly affected.

324 Glasser's disease A pig with meningitis. Note the evidence of paddling movements with its limbs.

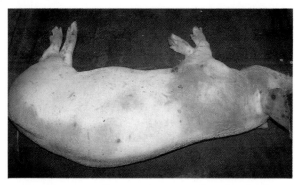

325 Glasser's disease Carcase of a pig which has died from Glasser's disease. Note the cyanosis of the extremities and the focal skin lesions.

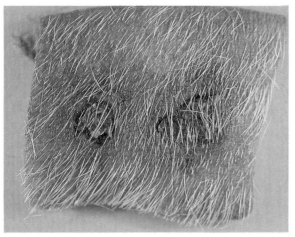

326 Glasser's disease Close up of the skin lesions from the pig shown in **325**.

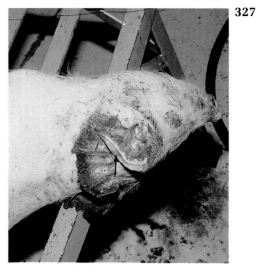

327 Glasser's disease Carcase of a 40 kg pig which died from Glasser's disease showing necrosis of the ears and the characteristic thickening of the pinna seen in many affected pigs (arrow).

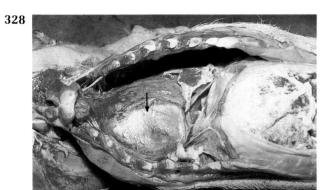

328 Glasser's disease Pleural cavity of a pig which died from Glasser's disease. There is fibrinous pericarditis (arrow) and fibrinous perihepatitis (right). The organism (*H. parasuis*) can be cultured from the lesions in early cases, but is more difficult to recover from chronic cases, or from pigs which have been treated.

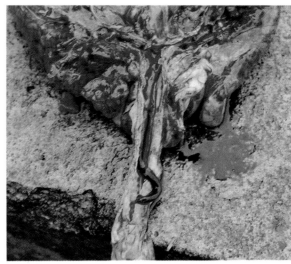

32

329 Glasser's disease Lungs from a 20 kg pig which had died from Glasser's disease. Note the clotted blood in the trachea, a feature sometimes seen in young pigs which have died from this disease.

Actinobacillus (Haemophilus) pleuropneumonia

Actinobacillus (Haemophilus) pleuro-pneumonia causes a pleuropneumonia in non-immune pigs of all ages and, in infected herds, causes disease mainly from 8–10 weeks of age onwards. Affected pigs may die after a fever lasting a few hours, may recover from the acute disease completely or become chronically infected, with exercise intolerance and poor growth rates. The lesions of pleurisy and pneumonia persist until slaughter as abscesses in the lung and adhesions to the chest wall.

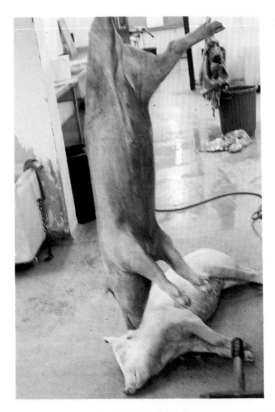

330 *Actinobacillus (H.) pleuropneumoniae*
The two 75 kg pigs shown here died suddenly from the disease. Note the congestion. Sudden death may also occur during transport or in lairage. The incubation period can be as short as 12 hours or even less.

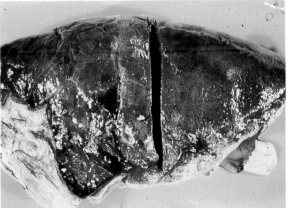

331 *Actinobacillus (H.) pleuropneumoniae*
Infected lung. Note the visceral pleurisy, consolidation and haemorrhage.

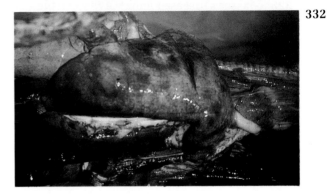

332 *Actinobacillus (H.) pleuropneumoniae*
Lung from an infected pig. Note the visceral pleurisy and haemorrhage around the necrotic lesions.

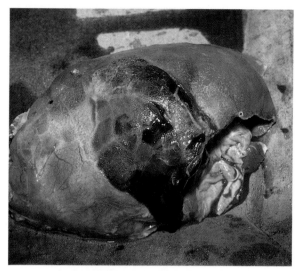

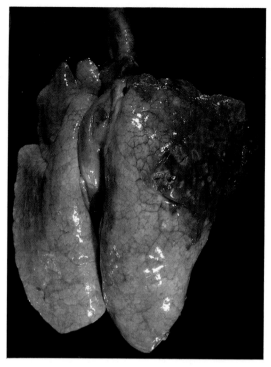

333 *Actinobacillus (H.) pleuropneumoniae*
Lungs from a 90 kg pig which had died from
pleuropneumonia caused by *A. (H.)
pleuropneumoniae*. A typical, well-
demarcated pneumonic lesion can be seen in
the proximal portion of the caudal lobe of the
left lung. The surfaces of the lesion and the
adjacent lung are covered by fibrin which in
older lesions becomes organised into fibrous
pleurisy. The organism can be isolated readily
from fresh lesions of this condition, but may
be more difficult to isolate from older lesions,
and from decaying tissue or when
antimicrobials have been given.

334 *Actinobacillus (H.) pleuropneumoniae*
Lungs from a pig killed 24 hours after
experimental inoculation with *A. (H.)
pleuropneumoniae*. The early lesions can be
clearly seen in the right lung and are marked
by pale areas of necrosis even after such a
short incubation period.

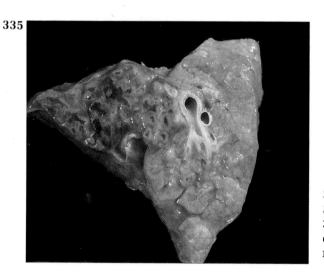

335 *Actinobacillus (H.) pleuropneumoniae*
Section through the early lesions shown in
334 to illustrate the consolidated appearance
of the affected lung. The unaffected lung is
much paler.

336 *Actinobacillus (H.) pleuropneumoniae*
Trachea from a natural case of
pleuropneumonia in a 20 kg pig opened to
display the purulent exudate which is seen in
some cases.

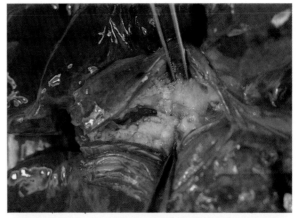

337 *Actinobacillus (H.) pleuropneumoniae*
Lungs from a 90 kg pig at slaughter in which
the chronic lesions can be seen. They appear
as bilateral multiple abscesses (arrows) and are
surrounded by fibrous adhesions which often
cause tearing of the lung at evisceration and
necessitate the stripping of the pleura.

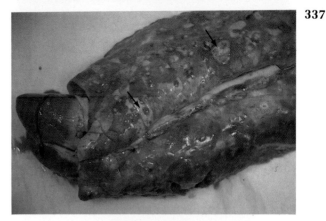

338 *Actinobacillus (H.) pleuropneumoniae*
The carcase of a finishing pig split to
demonstrate the extensive and severe pleurisy
that occurs in pleuropneumonia and which
frequently necessitates stripping of the pleura.

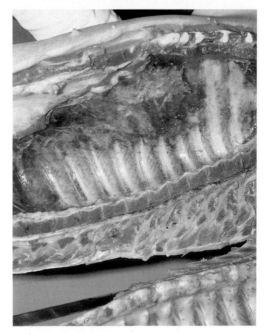

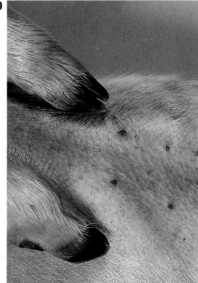

Escherichia coli Infections

Escherichia coli is both a normal inhabitant of the lower gastrointestinal tract of the pig and a cause of septicaemia, enteritis, mastitis, cystitis and other infectious conditions. The single species exists as many distinct strains, each with properties which allow it to survive harmlessly in the gut or to cause a particular disease syndrome in a non-immune pig. The ways in which they cause disease is known in considerable detail for some enteric strains, but less is known about those associated with cystitis and mastitis. The photographs which follow illustrate the main syndromes associated with the organism.

E. coli septicaemia

Colisepticaemia occurs in neonatal piglets which have not ingested colostrum, or which have taken colostrum containing little or no antibody to the particular strain of *E. coli* present in the environment into which they are born. Piglets die within 1–2 days of birth after transient fever and increasing signs of weakness ending in convulsions and death. *E. coli* can be isolated from all parts of the carcase.

Lesions due to infection are rare or difficult to detect. Enteritis is often absent in uncomplicated cases. Histological sections often supplement the findings of bacteriological examination.

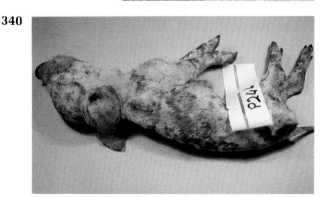

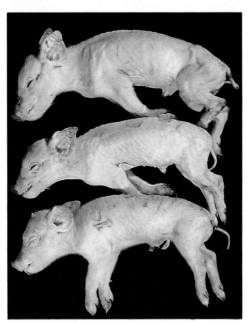

339 *Escherichia coli* **infection** Congested feet and nipples in a pig which died from *E. coli* septicaemia.

340 *Escherichia coli* **neonatal diarrhoea** Piglets which die from *E. coli* diarrhoea are often covered in diarrhoeic faeces from littermates as in the case of this one-day-old piglet.

341 *Escherichia coli* **neonatal diarrhoea** The three washed piglets shown here died from *E. coli* diarrhoea and are clearly dehydrated. Note how tightly the skin is drawn over the ribs and the prominence of the pelvic bones.

342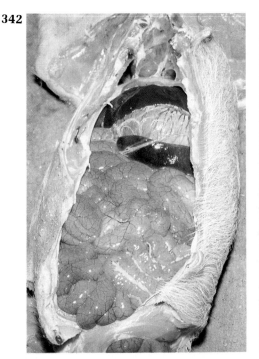

343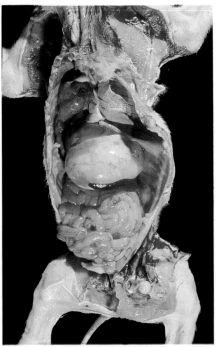

342 *Escherichia coli* neonatal diarrhoea The carcase of a two-day-old piglet which died from *E. coli* diarrhoea opened to demonstrate the pale, fluid-filled intestines. The hair coat is prominent because of the dehydration.

343 *Escherichia coli* neonatal diarrhoea The carcase of a two-day-old piglet which died from *E. coli* diarrhoea opened to show the dehydrated appearance of the internal organs and the distended stomach filled with milk. The intestines are filled with fluid but not inflamed.

44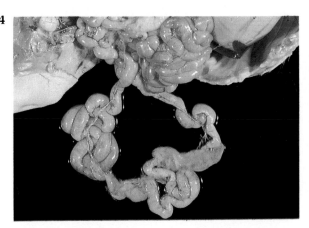

345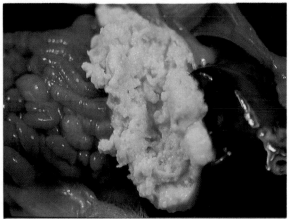

344 *Escherichia coli* neonatal diarrhoea The intestines of a two-day-old piglet which died from *E. coli* diarrhoea opened to show the pale, uninflamed mucosa and the pale contents seen in the uncomplicated disease.

345 *Escherichia coli* neonatal diarrhoea The milk clot in the stomach of affected piglets is frequently found to be laminated, as in this picture.

Escherichia coli Post-weaning Diarrhoea

Post-weaning diarrhoea due to *E. coli* commonly occurs 4–10 days after weaning. As milk antibody is withdrawn at weaning and as passive colostral immunity wanes, the pig can be infected with strains carrying the K88 antigen which have the ability to secrete heat labile enterotoxin (LT). Affected pigs develop watery or brownish diarrhoea and may die from dehydration. The carcases of these pigs often appear dehydrated with sunken eyes, prominent backbones and ribs and a hollow abdomen. The perineal region may be stained with diarrhoea and some dead pigs are in poor condition. Others die in good condition before diarrhoea develops.

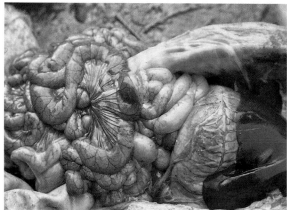

346 *Escherichia coli* post-weaning diarrhoea
This photograph is of a pig which died from post-weaning diarrhoea and illustrates the dark, dry liver, the stomach distended with food and the fluid-filled small intestines.

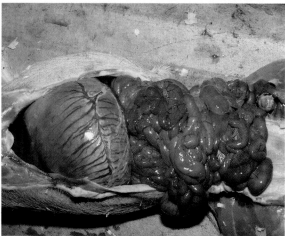

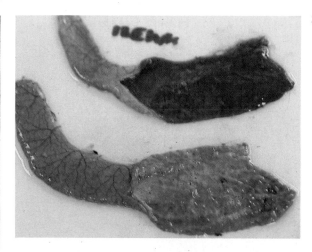

347 *Escherichia coli* post-weaning diarrhoea
The carcase of a pig which died from post-weaning *E. coli* diarrhoea demonstrating the degree of stomach filling sometimes seen, and the congestion of the small intestine often seen in these cases. The causal strain of *E. coli* can be isolated readily from the intestinal lumen but is rarely present in significant numbers in cultures made from other organs of fresh carcases.

348 *Escherichia coli* post-weaning diarrhoea
Ileums from two pigs which had died from *E. coli* post weaning diarrhoea opened to show the variation in degree of congestion from case to case.

349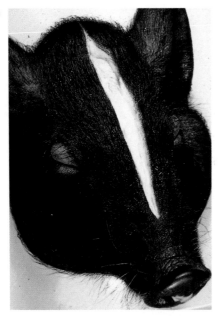

350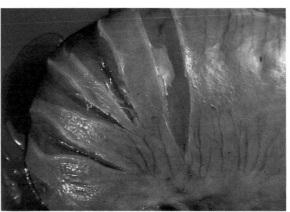

350 *Escherichia coli* bowel oedema The stomach from the pig shown in **349**. The wall has been cut to demonstrate the oedema. Fluid can be seen leaking from the incisions.

349 *Escherichia coli* bowel oedema (Oedema disease) The head of a pig which has recently died from bowel oedema. Note the puffy eyelids due to oedema and the subcutaneous oedema revealed by the incision.

351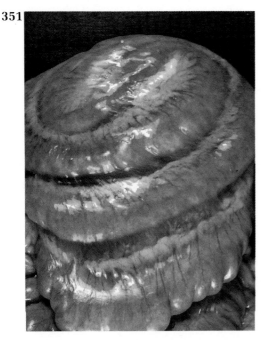

352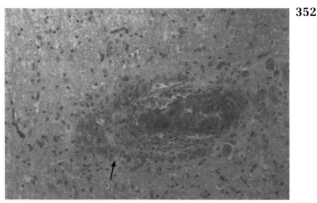

352 *Escherichia coli* bowel oedema When few or no gross lesions of oedema disease are visible, the diagnosis can be confirmed by histological means. The disease results from the effects of toxin on the medial region of arterial walls which become oedematous. The oedema is most prominent around cerebro spinal arteries and gives rise to cerebro spinal angiopathy, which is illustrated in this photograph. Note the proteinaceous fluid surrounding the artery and staining pink in this H and E photomicrograph (arrow).

351 *Escherichia coli* bowel oedema The spiral colon of the pig shown in **349**. Note the severe oedema of the mesentery.

353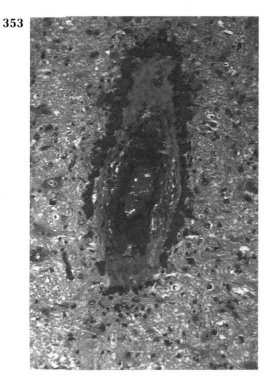

354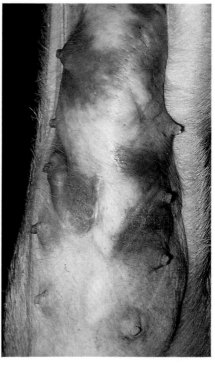

353 *Escherichia coli* bowel oedema A photomicrograph of cerebro spinal angiopathy stained to demonstrate disruption of the elastin layers of the arterial media (stained blue).

354 *Escherichia coli* mastitis Acute gangrenous mastitis resulting in death. Subacute forms are more common.

355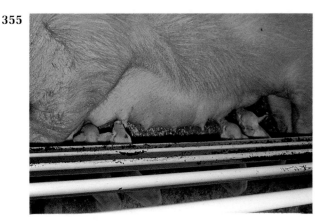

35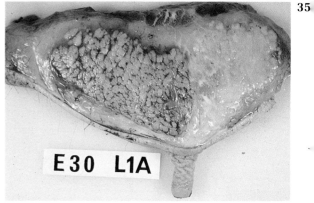

355 *Escherichia coli* mastitis An affected sow with two affected glands. The remainder of the udder is normal.

356 *Escherichia coli* mastitis The mammary glands have been sectioned to demonstrate the way in which only one gland is affected. The affected half is uniformly mottled and reddened, while the other half is normal.

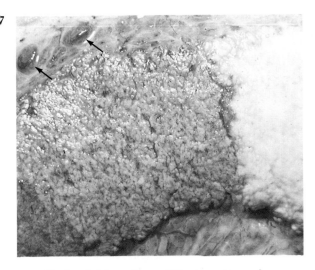

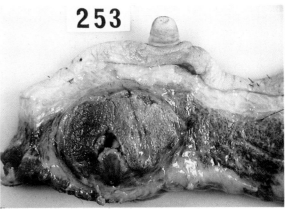

358 *Escherichia coli* **mastitis** An udder sectioned to show the damage caused by *E. coli* mastitis in a previous lactation.

357 *Escherichia coli* **mastitis** A section of an udder with gangrenous mastitis. Note the oedema, the enlarged lymph nodes (arrows) and the affected gland alongside a normal gland containing milk.

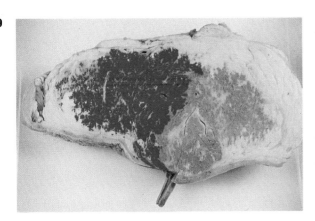

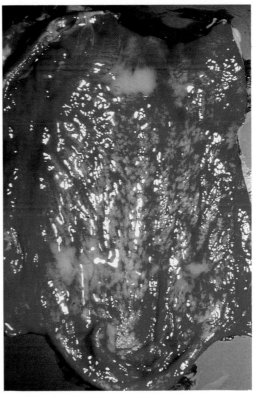

359 *Escherichia coli* **mastitis** A normal mammary gland in section. Yellow and red dyes have been injected into the teat canals to show that each mamma consists of two distinct subunits.

360 *Escherichia coli* **cystitis** The bladder from a five-year-old sow in the third month of pregnancy. Note the intensely reddened mucosa and the pools of pus resulting from acute coliform cystitis.

361

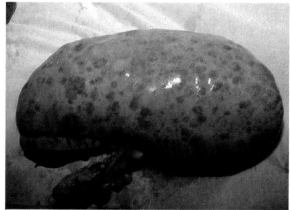

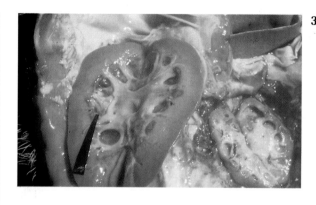

361 *Escherichia coli* pyelonephritis A kidney from the five-year-old sow with cystitis. There is an acute coliform pyelonephritis. Note the mottled surface of the kidney.

362 *Escherichia coli* pyelonephritis A kidney of a four-year-old sow opened to demonstrate the changes in pyelonephritis. Note the pus in the renal pelvis (indicated by the black strip).

363

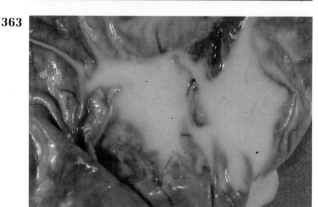

363 *Escherichia coli* metritis The uterus from a three-year-old sow which died from acute coliform metritis. Note the large quantities of yellow pus in the lumen.

364

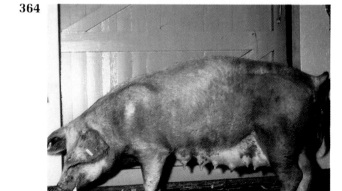

Klebsiella Infections

Klebsiella sp. can be isolated from chronic lesions of the respiratory tract, but are not the cause of any recognised syndrome.

364 *Klebsiella* mastitis *Klebsiella* mastitis resembles the acute form of *E. coli* mastitis clinically. Affected sows may die from systemic consequences. A severely affected sow is shown in this photograph. Note the purple discolouration of the flanks and the swelling of the mammae.

365 *Klebsiella* mastitis A sow with mastitis caused by *Klebsiella sp.* Note the purple discolouration and swelling of the mammae.

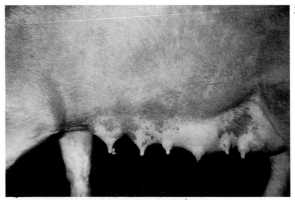

Leptospirosis

Leptospiral infections in pigs can cause fever, septicaemia, jaundice, nephritis, meningitis, abortion, infertility and death. A number of different serogroups are involved, with *Leptospira pomona* being most important worldwide, causing the most severe disease. In the UK, *L. canicola* may cause septicaemia and death in young pigs and *L. icterohaemorrhagiae* may cause both death and jaundice. Other serogroups such as *australis* and *hebdomadis* are involved in infertility and abortion.

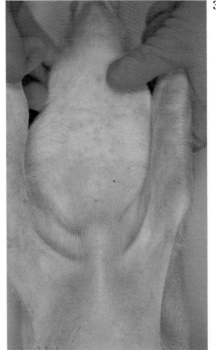

366

366 Leptospirosis Skin petechiation at the height of the septicaemic phase in *L. canicola* infection.

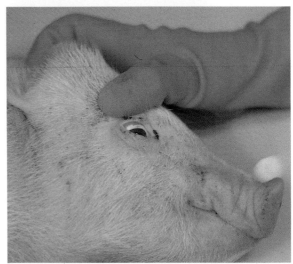

367

367 Leptospirosis *L. canicola* infection. Haemorrhages may be seen on the sclera of the eye.

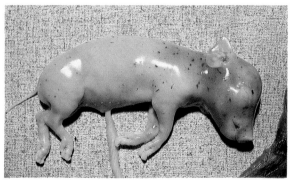

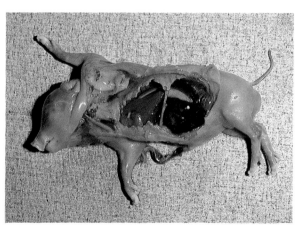

368 Leptospirosis Piglet from a late abortion caused by *L. pomona*. Note the skin haemorrhages. The thimbles on the claws are intact indicating that the piglet was born dead.

369 Leptospirosis *L. pomona*-infected foetus. The thoracic and abdominal cavities have been exposed. Note necrotic lesions in the liver.

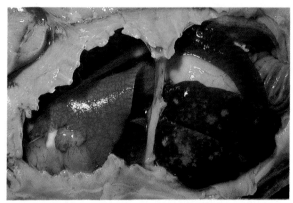

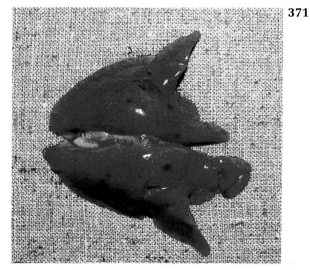

370 Leptospirosis *L. pomona* infection. Close-up of liver lesions. These are present in only a small proportion (less than 10 percent) of cases but are pathognomonic.

371 Leptospirosis *L. pomona* infection. Note the haemorrhages in the lungs of this aborted foetus.

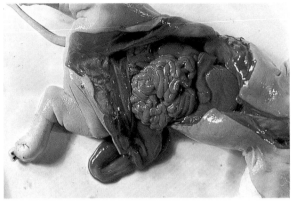

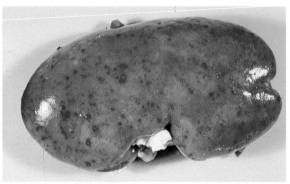

372 Leptospirosis A foetus aborted as a result of *L. canicola* infection. Both freshly aborted haemorrhagic foetuses, and those resembling that pictured here, may be found. In fresh material the organism may be demonstrated in foetal lung or liver by immunofluorescence or culture. In immunologically competent foetuses or stillborn piglets which have experienced intrauterine leptospiral infection, antibody may be demonstrated in pericardial, pleural and peritoneal fluid.

373 Leptospirosis Haemorrhages and petechiae occur throughout the body in pigs which have died or been killed in the acute phase of the disease. The focal haemorrhages in this kidney from a pig infected with *L. canicola* are typical.

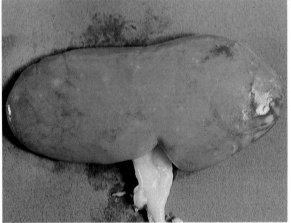

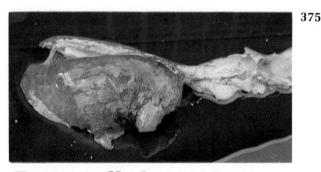

Pasteurella haemolytica

P. haemolytica can infect pigs to produce septicaemia in young animals and a pleuro-pneumonia-like condition in older pigs. In the UK, the infection has usually followed contact with sheep and is uncommon.

374 Leptospirosis A kidney from a chronic renal carrier of *L. canicola* in which small white foci of interstitial nephritis can be seen (arrows). This type of lesion is commonly found incidentally at slaughter. Such lesions are indicative of leptospiral infection and care should be taken by slaughterhouse workers when handling these cases. This also applies to *L. pomona* infection.

375 *Pasteurella haemolytica* The lungs shown here are from a seven-day-old piglet which died from *P. haemolytica* septicaemia. Type T organisms were recovered. Petechiae and haemorrhages were present on many organs, such as the kidney shown in **376**.

376

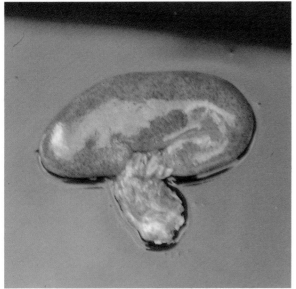

376 *Pasteurella haemolytica* A kidney from a seven-day-old piglet which died from *P. haemolytica* septicaemia. Note the petechiae.

Pasteurella multocida Pneumonia

P. multocida causes pneumonia in pigs of any age from weaning onwards. Affected pigs develop fever, raised respiratory rate and exercise intolerance. Severely affected animals may develop cyanosis of the extremities and die. Lesions are usually restricted to the lungs which are pneumonic, although some animals may have enlarged spleens.

377

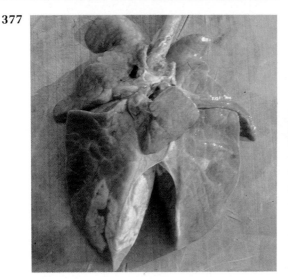

378

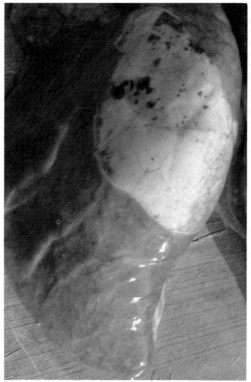

377 *Pasteurella multocida* pneumonia Lungs from a 10-week-old pig which died from *Pasteurella* pneumonia. All lobes in this ventral view are affected.

378 *Pasteurella multocida* pneumonia Dorsal surface of the left lung featured in **377** demonstrating the difference between a normal lung (arrow) and the lesions of pasteurellosis.

379 *Pasteurella multocida* pneumonia Cross-section through the pasteurellosis lesion shown in **378**. Note the complete consolidation of the lung and its pale colour, which is due to accumulations of fibrin and inflammatory cells in the alveoli. *P. multocida* of types A and sometimes D can be isolated in pure culture.

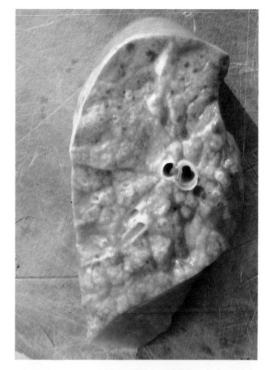

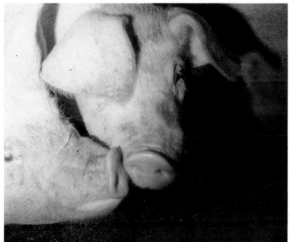

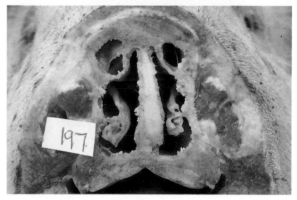

381 Toxin positive *Pasteurella multocida* type D Cross-section of the snout of a 10-week-old pig with atrophic rhinitis. Note the displaced septum and the atrophic ventral conchae. These lesions can be scored to give a measurement of the severity of the disease in a herd.

380 Toxin positive *Pasteurella multocida* type D Infection with this organism in neonatal non-immune piglets can result in the development of atrophic rhinitis when the toxin produced destroys the developing conchal bones of the nose. Inflammation causes bloody and serous nasal discharges and paroxysmal sneezing. Later in life atrophy and deviation of the snout occur.

This picture shows two pigs showing snout changes caused by *P. multocida* type D.

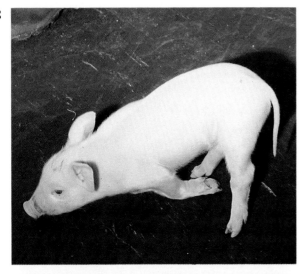

Streptococcus suis type I

S. suis type I is a cause of septicaemia, meningitis and arthritis most frequently in unweaned piglets. Infection is carried by the sow and invades the tonsils of unprotected piglets to cause fever and death in some cases. Other members of the litter may develop the less severe clinical signs. Arthritis acquired by five to 10 days of age can depress productivity and affect pigs until much later in life. The organism can be isolated readily from carcases of piglets that have died in the septicaemic stage, or from the brains and joints of those with meningitis and arthritis.

382 *Streptococcus suis* type I The piglet shown here was two weeks old and had such severe streptococcal arthritis it was unable to stand.

Streptococcus suis type II

S. suis type II is a frequent cause of streptococcal meningitis in pig herds. The organism may cause septicaemia but the main clinical signs are those of meningitis in weaned pigs up to 60 kg liveweight, although non-immune adults can also be affected. Affected pigs are febrile, appear glassy-eyed, may have tremor of the head, convulsions and may die within hours or survive with clinical signs for several days. Survivors may be left with permanent brain damage.

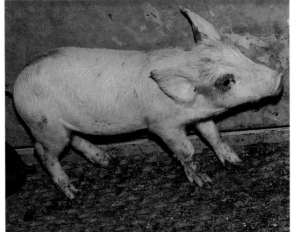

383 *Streptococcus suis* type II A piglet in the early stages of the disease. Note the slight tilting of the head.

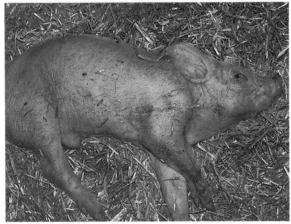

384 *Streptococcus suis* type II A pig with meningitis. Affected pigs may remain in this state even after apparently successful antimicrobial treatment and recover only gradually.

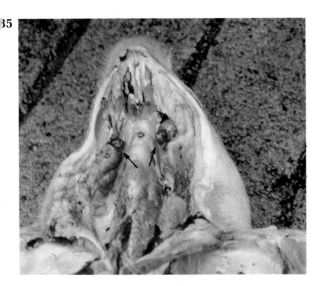

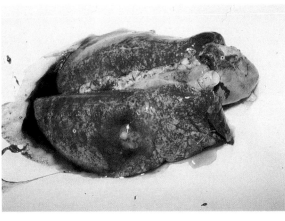

385 *Streptococcus suis* **type II** Congestion of the lymph nodes is common in animals which have died from acute *S. suis* type II infection. Here, an affected pig has been dissected to demonstrate the submandibular lymph nodes (arrow).

386 *Streptococcus suis* **type II** The lungs from a 20 kg weaner with *S. suis* type II septicaemia. Note the oedema and multiple petechial haemorrhages. A localised abscess is also present on the right lung. No *A. (H.) pleuropneumoniae* was present in the herd.

387 *Streptococcus suis* **type II** The brain may be congested in cases of streptococcal meningitis and at times accumulations of pus may be seen on the surface. On other occasions there may be no gross lesions. In most cases, the streptococcus responsible may be isolated from the brain in pure culture. Treatment prior to death may make this difficult.

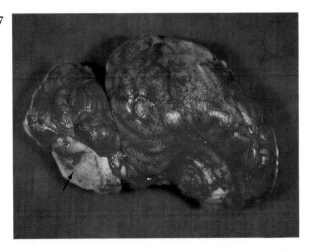

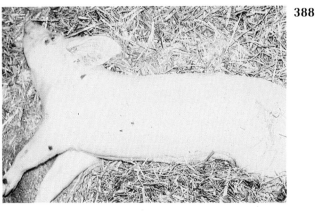

The brain shown here is acutely congested and the meningeal vessels are prominent. There is an accumulation of pus at the base of the cerebellum (arrow).

388 *Streptococcus suis* **type II** Live affected weaner. Note opisthotonus and paddling movements of front legs. These movements frequently lead to skin abrasions and bony prominences.

Salmonellosis

Several species of *Salmonella* infect the pig, but the majority cause no clinical disease. Some like *S. typhimurium* and *S. derby*, may cause fever and enteritis or enteritis alone and *S. dublin* may cause meningitis. *S. choleraesuis*, in particular, causes acute disease and death mainly in pigs 10 to 16 weeks old. The syndrome produced may be an acute septicaemia with sudden death and congestion of the extremities, or fever, pneumonia and diarrhoea containing shreds of necrotic material. In chronically affected pigs the extremities can become necrotic and may drop off.

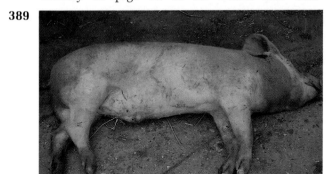

389 *Salmonella cholerasuis* Septicaemic form of *S. choleraesuis* infection. Note the cyanosis of the extremities and faecal soiling below anus.

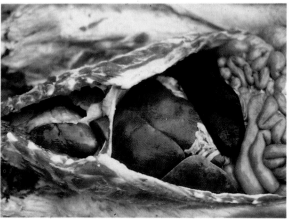

390 *Salmonella choleraesuis* The carcase of the pig shown in **389** opened to demonstrate the enlarged, friable, engorged spleen and fevered carcase.

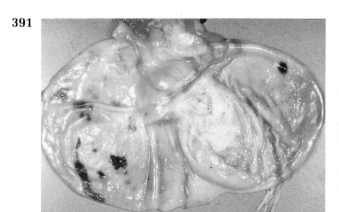

391 *Salmonella choleraesuis* The stomach from a case of salmonellosis showing haemorrhages in the gastric mucosa and at the pylorus.

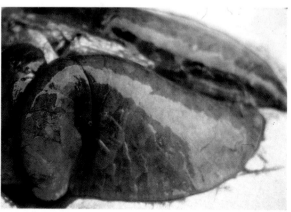

392 *Salmonella choleraesuis* Lungs from a pig which died from *S. choleraesuis* septicaemia. Note the congestion.

393 *Salmonella typhimurium* An acute case with intestinal haemorrhage resulting in death.

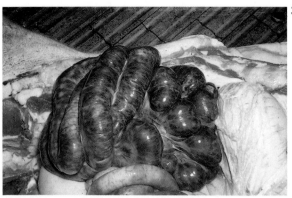

Exudative Epidermitis (Greasy Pig Disease)

Staphylococcus hyicus causes Exudative Epidermitis or Greasy Pig Disease, a syndrome seen in piglets aged from seven days to 10 weeks. In sucking piglets the disease may be acute, but as piglets grow older the more chronic form of the disease is likely to be seen. In acute cases a marked inflammation of the skin occurs followed by exudation of fluid.

Affected piglets develop brownish scales and crusts which rapidly spread to involve the whole surface of the body. The piglets lose condition, appear very hairy and are covered with a greasy exudate. Affected piglets may die rapidly from dehydration, recover slowly or remain stunted for some weeks.

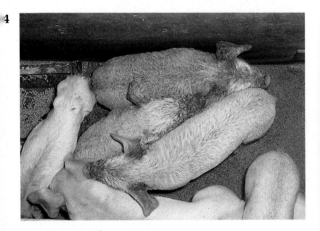

394 Exudative epidermitis An affected litter of piglets with both severely diseased animals and normal litter mates.

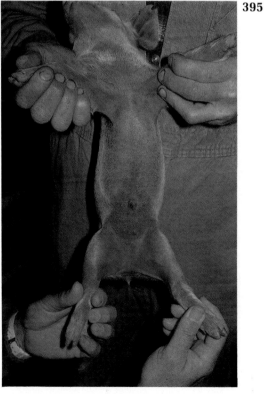

395 Exudative epidermitis Early disease with marked inflammation of skin.

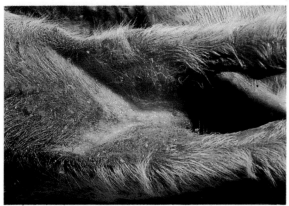

396 Exudative epidermitis Lesions of generalised acute exudative epidermitis. Note the moist appearance of the axillae and the colour of the skin.

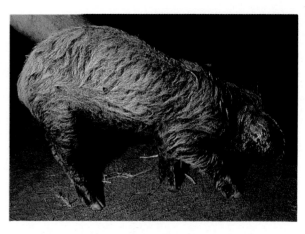

397 Exudative epidermitis A severely affected weaner seven days after the onset of the condition.

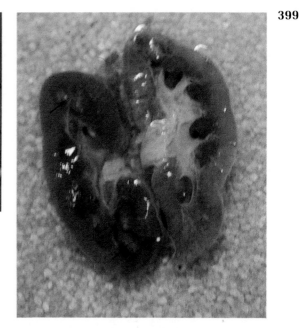

398 Exudative epidermitis A subacute case with multifocal lesions.

399 Exudative epidermitis Post-mortem lesions of exudative epidermitis are mainly restricted to the skin and draining lymph nodes which are thickened or enlarged. Other organs are affected by dehydration and changes are most prominent in the kidney where urate crystals are deposited in the medulla, as shown in this photograph (see arrow).

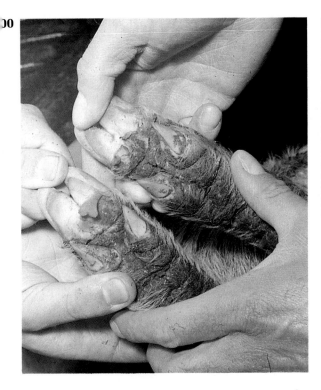

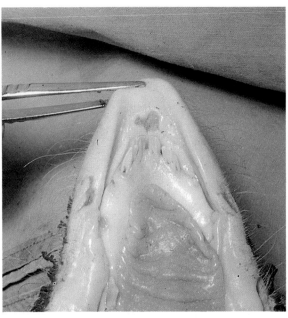

401 Exudative epidermitis Mouth lesions in an affected piglet.

400 Exudative epidermitis Foot lesions. Note the lesions on the bulbs of the heels.

Exudative Epidermitis – Adults

S. hyicus infections in adults are more localised and less commonly identified. They vary between patches of skin covered in exudate to multifocal pyoderma with ulceration. The following series of photographs illustrates these lesions.

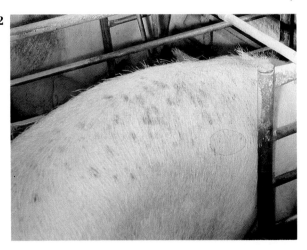

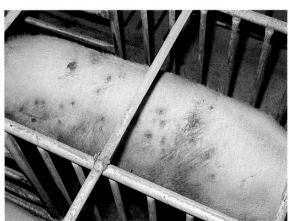

403 Exudative epidermitis Widespread multifocal pyoderma with ulceration.

402 Exudative epidermitis Early localised lesions without ulceration.

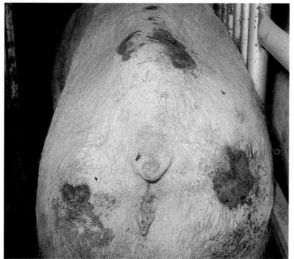

404 Exudative epidermitis Close-up of extensive acute lesions of multifocal pyoderma.

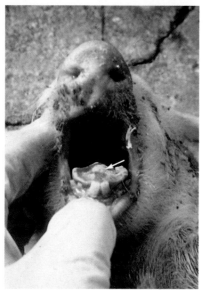

Fusobacterium necrophorum and Necrotic Stomatitis

F. necrophorum is involved in many syndromes in which necrosis of tissues occurs. This anaerobe produces powerful necrotising toxins. It is particularly associated with necrotic stomatitis initiated by tooth clipping. Affected pigs suck with difficulty, lose condition and die. Fight wounds may also be infected.

405 Lesions of necrotic stomatitis. Necrotic material is present on the tongue (arrow). Note the poor condition of the piglet.

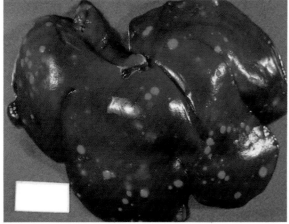

406 *Fusobacterium necrophorum* infection Liver showing multiple abscesses. Smears made from these necrotic areas usually contain large numbers of the long, thin, beaded Gram-negative rods.

Treponema hyodysenteriae Infection (Swine Dysentery)

Infection with *T. hyodysenteriae* causes swine dysentery, a mucohaemorrhagic diarrhoea of weaned pigs resulting in loss of condition, depression of growth rate and, in severe cases, death. The clinical signs are pathognomonic and consist of a blood-stained diarrhoea containing mucus.

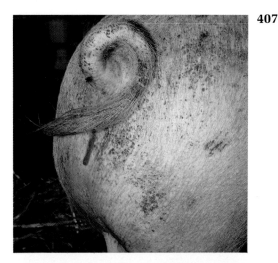

407 *Treponema hyodysenteriae* **infection (swine dysentery)** The hindquarters of a pig with classic swine dysentery. Note the trickle of blood-stained diarrhoea.

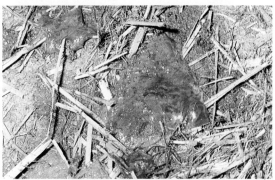

408 *Treponema hyodysenteriae* **infection (swine dysentery)** Blood-stained mucoid faeces from a case of swine dysentery. *T. hyodysenteriae* may be seen as a Gram-negative spirochaete in smears made from the faeces and isolated under anaerobic conditions.

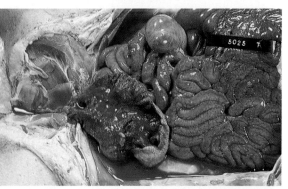

409 *Treponema hyodysenteriae* **infection (swine dysentery)** Pigs which die from swine dysentery are usually dehydrated and have intestinal lesions restricted to the large intestine. The other organs are usually unaffected although there may be congestion of the small intestine.

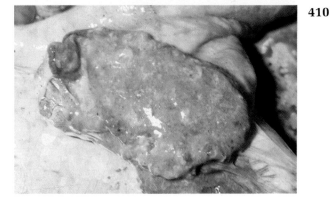

410 *Treponema hyodysenteriae* **infection (swine dysentery)** A portion of large intestine opened to show the mucoid nature of the contents. There is thickening of the large intestinal mucosa.

411

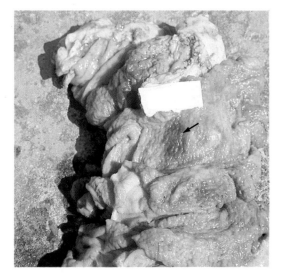

411 *Treponema hyodysenteriae* **infection (swine dysentery)** Washed colonic mucosa from a clinically normal recovered case of swine dysentery, showing a residual lesion of the disease (arrow).

Spirochaetal Diarrhoea

Spirochaetes which differ from *T. hyodysenteriae* are capable of infecting the large intestinal mucosa in non-immune pigs and when other agents such as nematodes or bacteria disrupt the epithelium. The infections cause mild colonic inflammation which is less severe than that caused by swine dysentery, but which allows the development of diarrhoea. Affected pigs rarely die, but pass a watery or pasty mucoid diarrhoea for several days accompanied by a marked loss in condition. Pigs are usually affected in the post-weaning period but the disease may occur in older animals.

412

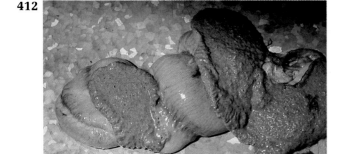

412 Spirochaetal diarrhoea The colon of a pig killed 11 days after infection with a non-*T. hyodysenteriae* spirochaete showing the dilatation of the organ but little inflammation.

41

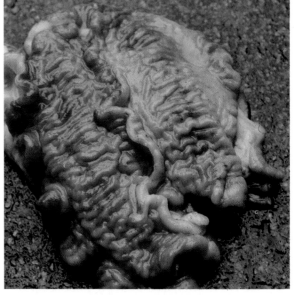

413 Spirochaetal diarrhoea Colonic mucosa washed to show the inflamed surface resulting from the spirochaetal infection.

414

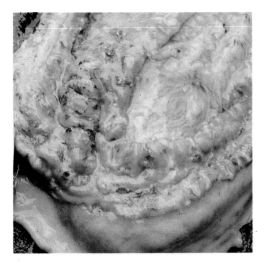

414 Spirochaetal diarrhoea Chronically-affected mucosa from a case of spirochaetal diarrhoea. Note the localised areas of necrotic debris which have formed over bleeding points such as those seen in the previous picture. These small necrotic particles may sediment out of colonic contents or faeces suspended in water.

415

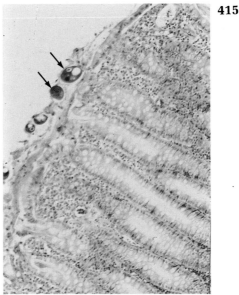

415 Spirochaetal diarrhoea A photomicrograph of the colonic mucosa of a case of spirochaetal diarrhoea showing dilated crypts and an accumulation of *Balantidium coli* on the surface (arrow).

Tuberculosis

Tuberculosis in the pig may be generalised when caused by *Mycobacterium bovis* and *M. intracellulare*, but the vast majority of infections are localised in the submandibular lymph nodes and are caused by avian tubercle bacteria (*M. avium*).

416

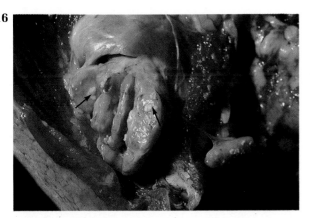

416 Tuberculosis A pig's head split in the course of carcase preparation is shown above. The lymph nodes have been exposed and cut to display the calcified granulomatous lesions of avian tuberculosis (arrow).

417

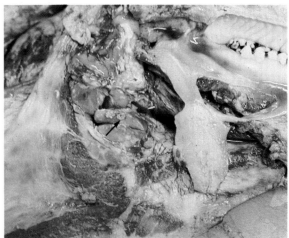

417 Tuberculosis A submandibular lymph node cut to demonstrate granulomas caused by *Mycobacterium intracellulare* (arrows).

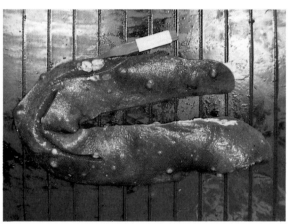

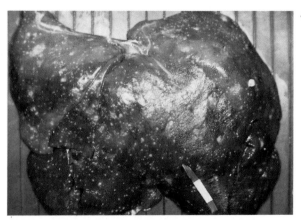

418 Tuberculosis Spleen from a pig with *M. bovis* infection. The granulomas appear as masses in the spleen or as white nodules. Their spherical nature is demonstrated in the two granulomas exposed by the cut.

419 Tuberculosis *M. bovis* causes systemic infection which may be seen as miliary granulomas throughout the liver and other organs. The white foci on the liver shown here are small (1–5 mm) tubercular granulomas.

Septic Omphalophlebitis (Navel Ill)

Infection of the navel cord commonly occurs within a short period (1–2 days) of birth. A number of bacteria may be responsible and infection may immediately spread to cause neonatal septicaemia and death. However, infection usually remains localised at the site of entry to produce an abscess. Abscesses become detectable at 5–10 days of age as swellings at the junction of the umbilical cord and the abdominal wall. In most cases this is visible externally, but occasionally the abscess can only be detected at post mortem examination. Affected pigs are fevered, anorexic and appear depressed. The abscess may resemble an umbilical hernia but is not reducible.

420

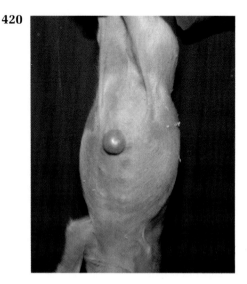

420 Septic omphalophlebitis (Navel Ill) An abscess visible from the exterior is shown on the ventral abdomen of this two-week-old piglet.

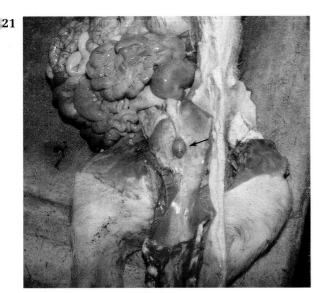

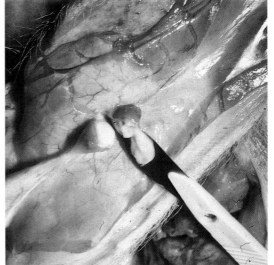

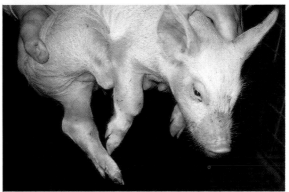

421 Septic omphalophlebitis (Navel Ill) A two-week-old piglet opened to show the abscess on the lateral or peritoneal surface (arrow).

422 Septic omphalophlebitis (Navel Ill) The piglet shown in **421**. The abscess has been excised to expose the thick creamy pus.

423 Septic omphalophlebitis (Navel Ill) A two-week-old piglet with both navel ill and joint ill. Both knee and hock joints are affected.

424 *Chlamydia psittaci* infection Chlamydial infections are rarely diagnosed, but the organism has been isolated from the uterus, vagina, arthritic joints, demonstrated in the intestinal mucosa and isolated from the respiratory tract. Respiratory infection is perhaps the most easily-recognised form of the disease because of the distribution of the lung lesions.

These lung lesions were produced by experimental infection with *C. psittaci*. Note the distribution of the lesions in the dorsal part of the caudal lobes of this set of lungs.

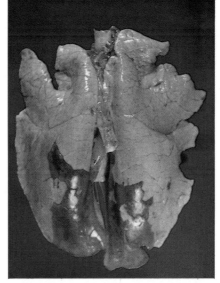

Mycoplasma hyopneumoniae Infection (Enzootic Pneumonia)

M. hyopneumoniae infects the respiratory tract of the pig and can initiate a pneumonia with a characteristic anterior lobe distribution known as Enzootic Pneumonia of Pigs (EPP). The disease has been identified worldwide and is a major cause of economic loss. Infection may not result in overt disease, as immunity, climate, the physical and social environment, and the presence of other respiratory pathogens all influence its development. In herds where the disease is enzootic, it is seen most commonly in weaned pigs following loss of maternal immunity and usually occurs in growing and finishing pigs (10–20 weeks of age). The clinical signs are coughing and uneven growth. More severe respiratory disease may occur in pigs of all ages following the introduction of infection into non-immune herds, but this is not always the case, and infection may be inapparent for months.

The infection may be complicated and made more severe by infection with other agents such as *Pasteurella multocida, Haemophilus* spp. and viruses such as influenza. The extent of the pneumonic lesions provides a guide to the economic importance of the disease within a herd. Lesions occupying 10 per cent or more of the lung are usually considered to reduce growth rate. The extent of lung lesions seen at slaughter may not reflect the severity of the disease in a herd because partial resolution has occurred.

The disease may be suspected in the live animal but confirmation of the disease requires the examination of lungs at slaughter. The histological appearance of the affected lung provides additional evidence (see below) and demonstration of the organism by its morphological appearance in Giemsa-stained smears, by immunofluorescence or, best of all, by culture confirms the presence of *M. hyopneumoniae*.

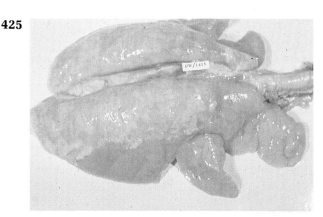

425 *Mycoplasma hyopneumoniae* Lungs from a field case of Enzootic Pneumonia uncomplicated by secondary bacterial infection. Note the typical distribution of the lesions in the cranial, cardiac and anteroventral caudal lobes.

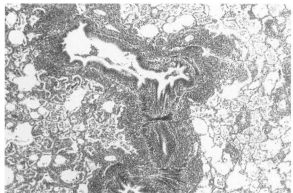

426 *Mycoplasma hyopneumoniae* (Enzootic Pneumonia) Histological section through a lesion 3½ months after experimental infection of a SPF (Specific Pathogen Free) pig with a pure culture of *M. hyopneumoniae* "J" strain. Note the massive cellular accumulations (stained purple).

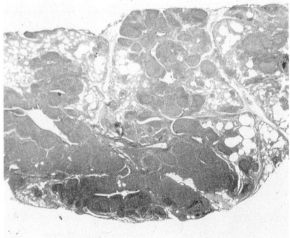

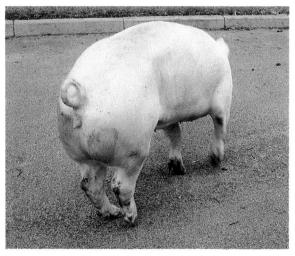

427 *Mycoplasma hyopneumoniae* infection **(Enzootic Pneumonia)** A histological section through an early lesion of Enzootic Pneumonia to demonstrate the typical peribronchial distribution of the lesions, 22 days after experimental infection with *M. hyopneumoniae* "J" strain.

428 *Mycoplasma hyosynoviae* A typical case of an infected first litter gilt. There is bilateral infection of both stifle and hock joints. Note the typical posture of an affected animal.

Mycoplasma hyosynoviae

Mycoplasma hyosynoviae causes synovitis and lameness in pigs. The disease is most commonly seen in large finishing pigs and young breeding stock. It is particularly important in the latter if it develops shortly after purchase, as it may have been bought in with the breeding animals or represent infection acquired after entry.

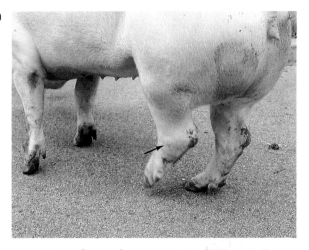

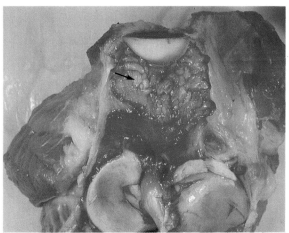

429 *Mycoplasma hyosynoviae* Mildly swollen hock joint (arrow) of the left hind leg of a lame maiden gilt.

430 *Mycoplasma hyosynoviae* A joint opened to show the marked villous hypertrophy of the synovial membrane (arrow).

431

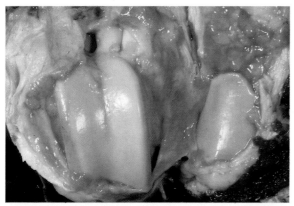

431 *Mycoplasma hyosynoviae* A stifle joint showing synovitis and pannus formation.

432

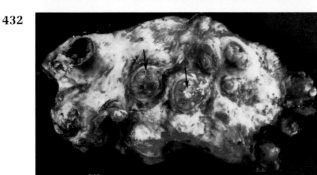

432 'Actinomycosis' of the udder Large granulomatous areas in the udder which ulcerate to discharge yellowish pus are often attributed to 'actinomycosis'. Investigation often reveals the presence of bacteria but *Actinomyces* spp. are rarely isolated. The affected mammary gland shown here has had the skin removed to show the large granulomas (arrows).

433

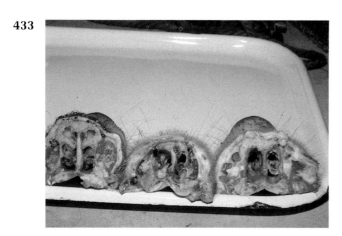

433 Atrophic Rhinitis Atrophic Rhinitis is an infectious disease of young actively growing pigs. After sneezing and other signs of upper respiratory tract infection, shortening and, sometimes, twisting of the snout occurs by 6–8 weeks of age. Section of the snout between first and second premolars allows the extent of the lesions to be seen clearly. These lesions can be subjectively graded on a scale of 0–5 (*see* **381**).

This photograph shows the snouts from three 20 kg weaners, sectioned to show varying degrees of atrophy.

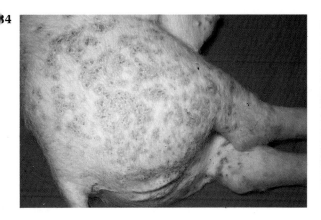

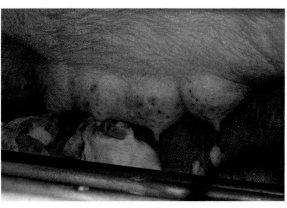

434 Staphylococcal infection Staphylococcal acne in the offspring of hysterectomy-derived sows.

435 Staphylococcal infection Note the microabscesses on the udder of a recently-farrowed sow. Staphylococci were cultured (*see also* **160**).

Viral Diseases

Porcine Parvovirus infection

Parvoviruses are small, resistant DNA viruses and multiply best in rapidly-dividing tissues. In the pig, they multiply in the cells of the conceptus and kill the foetuses of non-immune sows in the period prior to the development of immunocompetence at around 67 days of gesta-

436

tion. These dead foetuses become mummified. Infection may spread along uterine horns, gradually affecting each foetus in turn. Older affected foetuses may be stillborn.

436 Porcine parvovirus infection In this photograph, a series of stillborn piglets is seen. The smallest piglets died first and the largest last; most of the mummified piglets died prior to 70 days gestation and the pale piglets died prior to parturition or during it.

Virus antigen can usually be demonstrated in the lung and liver tissue of mummified piglets but cannot be demonstrated in the stillborn animals. Antibody to porcine parvovirus can be demonstrated in the pleural and peritoneal transudates in the stillborn animals.

Polioencephalomyelitis

Infection with enteroviruses of Serogroup 1 strains can result in spread from the gut, which is the primary site of multiplication, to other parts of the body such as the central nervous system. The clinical syndrome associated with the most pathogenic strain of this serotype is known as Teschen disease and the disease and the virus are notifiable in many countries. Affected pigs develop fever, go off their feed and rapidly develop flaccid, usually posterior

paralysis and may die within three to four days. In some cases convulsions may be seen. Mild disease known as Talfan disease or Benign Enzootic Paresis may be caused by less pathogenic strains of the virus. Mortality is rare and affected pigs may only develop posterior paresis. In cases in which recovery occurs, muscle wasting may develop and persist, as motor neurones in the brain and spinal cord are destroyed by the virus.

437

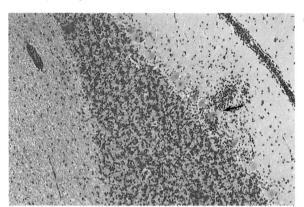

437 Teschen Disease A pig with Teschen disease. Note the position of the animal, with head back, paddling movements of the forelimbs and paresis of the hind limbs.

438 Polioencephalomyelitis The cerebellum of a pig which died from Talfan disease. There is loss of neurones and accumulations of microglial cells may be seen around some degenerating cells (arrow).

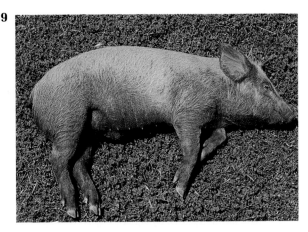

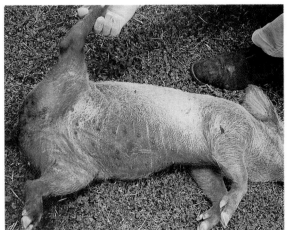

439 Encephalomyocarditis Sudden death with very severe cyanosis of the skin and the extremities. The disease is caused by encephalomyocarditis virus, a member of the cardiovirus group of enteroviruses. Viral antibodies have been detected in the UK but clinical disease has never been diagnosed.

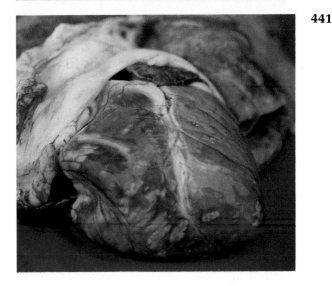

440 Encephalomyocarditis Note severe cyanosis of extremities.

441 Encephalomyocarditis Note the multiple necrotic lesions in the myocardium.

Transmissible Gastroenteritis (TGE)

Transmissible gastroenteritis is caused by a coronavirus which infects the mature epithelial cells at the tips of the villi of the small intestine. These are destroyed and villous atrophy results. This leads to profuse diarrhoea which is whitish in piglets or greenish grey in adults. Affected non-immune piglets under the age of three weeks may die from less severe dehydration although the widespread intro-duction of supplementary fluid for piglets has reduced mortality considerably.

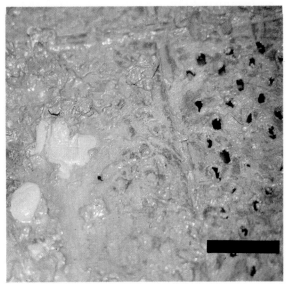

442 Transmissible Gastroenteritis Faeces in a pen containing a sow and litter with TGE. Note the greyish green colour and watery texture of most of the faeces and the soft white motion full of undigested milk fat passed by a recovering piglet.

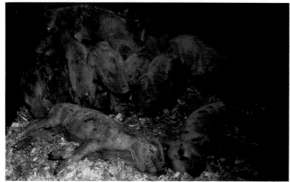

443 Transmissible Gastroenteritis Dying three-day-old piglets. Note the dehydration.

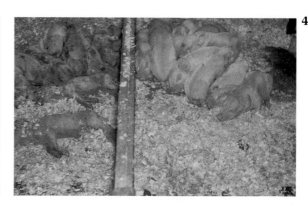

444 Transmissible Gastroenteritis Affected and non-affected three-day-old piglets. Note the good condition of the piglets on the right.

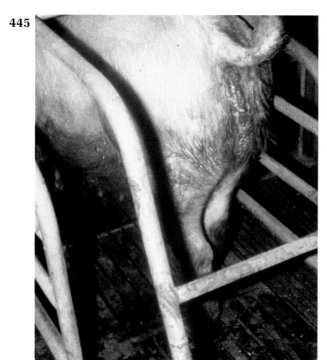

445 Transmissible Gastroenteritis An affected sow. Note the faecal staining of the perineum.

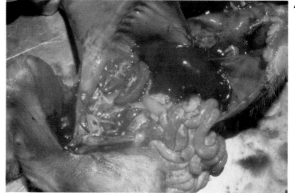

446 Transmissible Gastroenteritis Carcase of a four-day-old piglet opened to show the small intestines distended with fluid and milk clot.

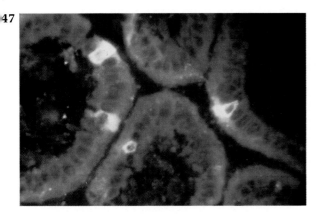

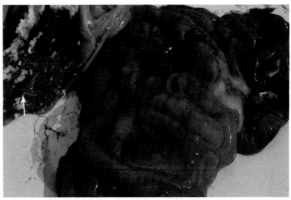

447 Transmissible Gastroenteritis Frozen section of the small intestine of a piglet with TGE. It has been stained with fluorescent antibody to the virus, the test used widely to confirm infection. Infected cells fluoresce.

448 Epidemic Diarrhoea Type II Stomach and intestines from a piglet with Epidemic Diarrhoea. Note the congested gastric mucosa (arrow) and the distended, fluid-filled small intestine.

Rotavirus Infection

Rotaviruses also multiply in the intestinal epithelial cells to cause cell shedding and loss of absorptive capacity. Diarrhoea results in many cases and may occur in both sucking piglets and in weaned pigs. In most cases, the disease occurs in individual pigs and not as an epidemic, but the virus will infect all individuals at some stage or other. The post mortem findings are similar to those of Epidemic Diarrhoea Type II.

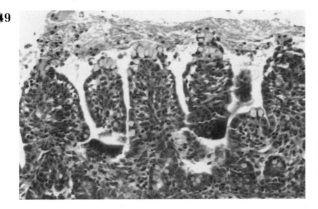

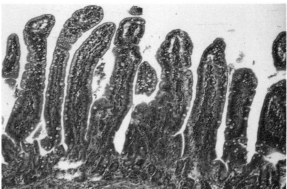

449 Rotavirus infection Histological section of affected intestinal mucosa from a two-week-old piglet affected by rotaviral diarrhoea. Note the short villi and the loss of mature absorptive cells from the villous tips. The villi form a marked contrast with the normal villi shown in **450**.

450 Normal Intestinal Mucosa Histological section of villi from a normal pig of the same age as the one with rotavirus infection shown in **449**. Note the long thin villi.

Inclusion Body Rhinitis (IBR)

Infection with this cytomegalovirus usually occurs in early life and causes rhinitis which is rarely fatal except in very young pigs. Clinical signs of anorexia and mild pyrexia with occasional rhinitis occur from about three weeks of age onwards in piglets born to immune sows. Mild rhinitis may be seen at post mortem examination and characteristic histological lesions of cytomegaly and the presence of prominent intranuclear inclusions can be found in the cells of the glands of the nasal mucosa.

A more severe syndrome in which severe rhinitis, sneezing and deaths of up to 25 percent of piglets can occur in non immune piglets, after particularly early, or in utero infection. More extensive lesions are seen in these piglets, with oedema of the lungs, widespread serous effusions and haemorrhages, particularly of the kidney. Anaemia may also occur. Diagnosis is usually based on the presence of the characteristic inclusion bodies in affected tissue.

451

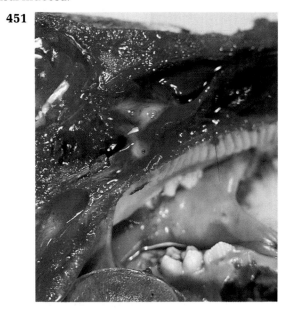

451 Inclusion Body Rhinitis A longitudinal section of the snout of a 12-day-old piglet illustrating the acute congestion of the conchal epithelium found in early cases of IBR.

452

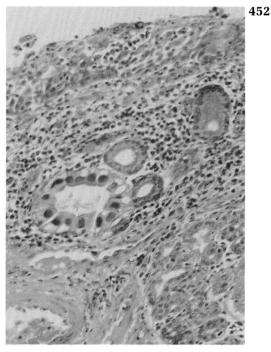

452 Inclusion Body Rhinitis Histological section of nasal mucosa showing the characteristic intranuclear bodies in the epithelial cells of the mucosal glands. Affected cells are markedly enlarged (when compared with those of the unaffected glandular tissue nearby). Note the inflammatory cells surrounding the affected gland.

Aujeszky's Disease (Pseudo Rabies)

This disease is caused by suid herpesvirus I which results in upper respiratory signs in older pigs and abortion in sows. In young piglets it frequently causes death associated with the development of nervous signs. Weaned and finishing pigs are less likely to die but depression of growth may be seen and pneumonia may occur. Infection in immune or partially immune herds may be inapparent. Recovered animals develop serum antibody in most cases, but may be latent carriers of the virus for life as the herpes virus is capable of integrating into the genome of cells such as those of the cranial nerve ganglia.

453 Aujeszky's Disease Piglet showing typical nervous signs just before its death. Affected piglets are often pyrexic (to 41.5°C, 107°F) and die in convulsions within 12 hours of the development of clinical signs. Note the outstretched forelimbs.

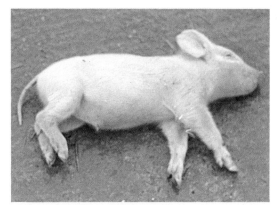

453

454 Aujeszky's Disease Dead piglets collected during an outbreak of Aujeszky's Disease in a 270 sow herd. Note the numbers involved and their uniformly small size. They are accompanied by the farm cat. The death of other species often draws attention to the presence of the disease on a pig farm, particularly as the clinical signs in these other species may be dramatic.

455 Aujeszky's Disease The head of a piglet showing the skin lesions sometimes seen on affected piglets.

456 Aujeszky's Disease The head of a piglet illustrating lesions present on the snout and palate (arrows).

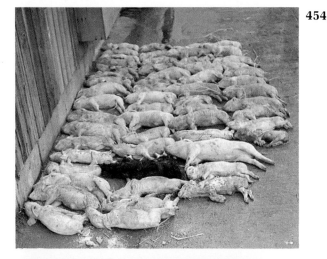

454

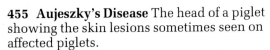

55

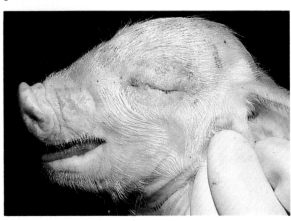

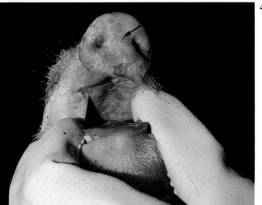

456

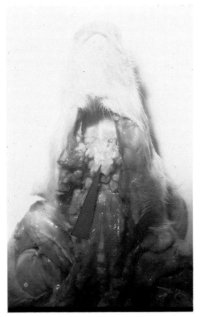

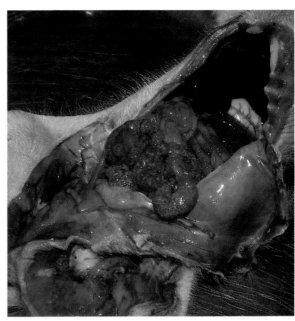

457 Aujeszky's Disease Post mortem picture
of a piglet demonstrating the presence of a
necrotic, diphtheritic membrane on the tonsils
(arrow). This is a common lesion.

458 Aujeszky's Disease Carcase opened to
demonstrate necrotic lesions in the wall of the
small intestine. These may also be seen in the
liver.

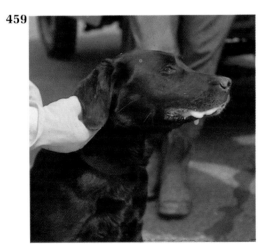

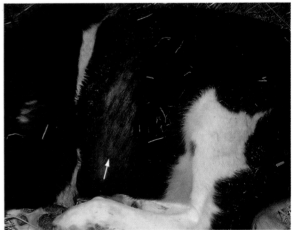

459 Aujeszky's Disease A dog salivating at the
mouth. This animal died within 24 hours.
Confirmation of Aujeszky's Disease was not
made but the animal was known to have eaten
piglets which had died on a farm where
Aujeszky's Disease was active. The disease is
dramatic and could be confused with rabies.

460 Aujeszky's Disease A six-month-old
Friesian calf with Aujeszky's Disease
following airspace contact with affected pigs.
Affected cattle often develop severe pruritis
and self-inflicted injuries are common. This
calf shows such lesions over the ribs (arrow).

Classical Swine Fever (Hog Cholera)

This is a highly contagious viral disease caused by a Pestivirus. It is characterised by its rapid spread, fever, high morbidity and mortality in susceptible herds, and by haemorragic lesions in many parts of the carcase. The disease has a worldwide distribution, but has been eradicated from the UK, USA and other countries.

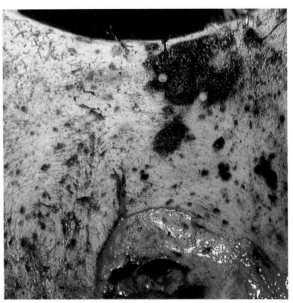

462 Swine Fever Marked haemorrhagic diathesis into the skin in the acute form of the disease.

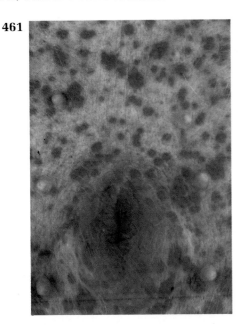

461 Classical Swine Fever (Hog Cholera) Haemorrhagic skin lesions in acute Swine Fever.

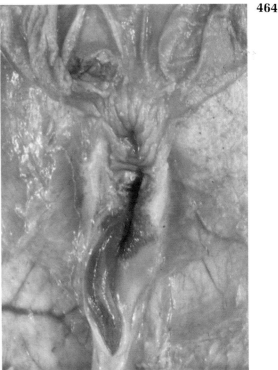

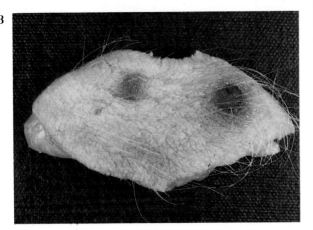

463 Swine Fever Chronic skin lesion (right). Note the necrotic centre of the lesion which will eventually be sloughed. The intensely congested tips of the ears and the tail may all be lost at this stage of the disease.

464 Swine Fever Haemorrhage in the preputial sac.

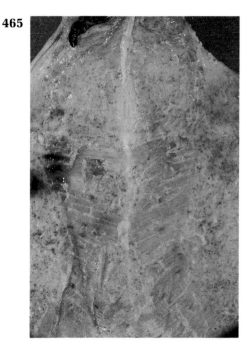

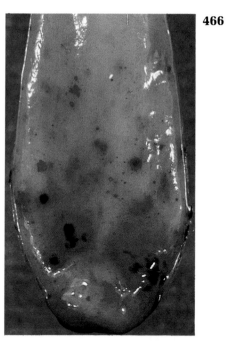

465 Swine Fever Haemorrhages and petechiation in the musculature.

466 Swine Fever Bladder from a case of acute Swine Fever. Note the areas of haemorrhage with dark, infarcted centres.

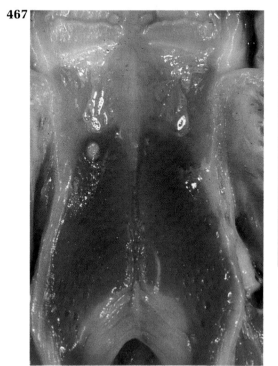

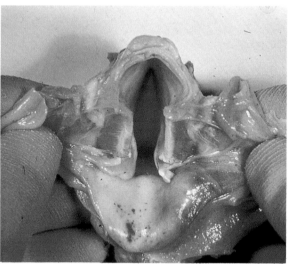

468 Swine Fever Haemorrhages on the epiglottis which are strongly suggestive of Swine Fever.

467 Swine Fever Tonsils from a case of acute Swine Fever. Note the congestion.

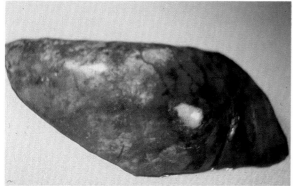

469 Swine Fever Lung from a case of Swine Fever. Note the haemorrhages. These may not appear in every case and may be complicated by the presence of other diseases.

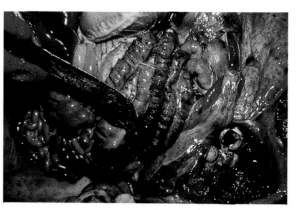

470 Swine Fever The abdominal viscera in an acute case.

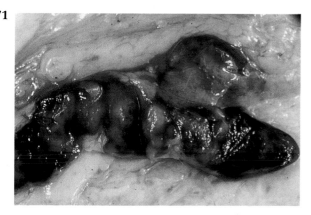

471 Swine Fever Mesenteric lymph nodes sectioned to show the typical subcapsular haemorrhages and their intensity.

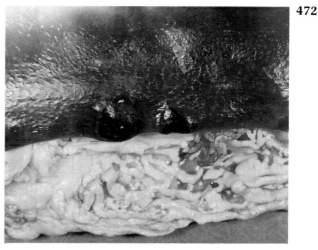

472 Swine Fever Infarction of the spleen occurs frequently in Swine Fever but rarely occurs in other diseases. Multiple infarcts may be present, usually along the margin as in this picture.

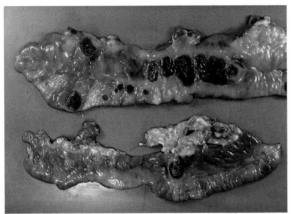

473 Swine Fever Lesions in the intestines may appear as prominent vessels in the serosal surface of the small intestine or as depressed circular areas in the serosal surface of the large intestine. These circular intestinal lesions develop into 'button ulcers' in chronic cases. They result from areas of infarction which become colonised by gut bacteria. These are early lesions in the large intestine of a pig with acute Swine Fever. Note their intensely haemorrhagic appearance.

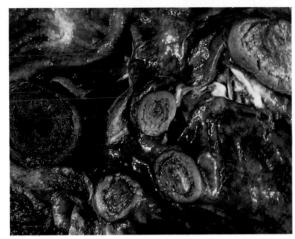

474 Swine Fever Large intestinal mucosa from a case of chronic Swine Fever. Note the well-defined circular areas of necrosis or 'button ulcers' which are pathognomonic of the disease.

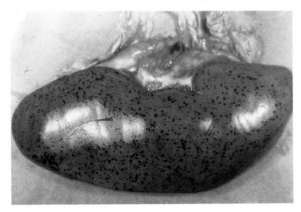

475 Swine Fever Surface of the kidney of an acute case of Swine Fever. The capsule of the kidney has been stripped to expose the petechiated surface. This 'turkey egg' kidney is present in many septicaemic conditions and is often present in this disease. When found, Swine Fever should be suspected.

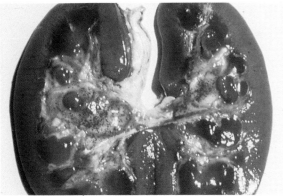

476 Swine Fever Haemorrhages in the pelvis of the kidney strongly suggestive of the disease.

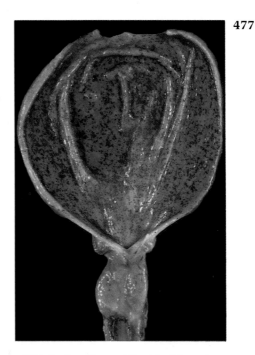

477 Swine Fever The bladder of an acute case of Swine Fever opened to show the petechiation of the cystic mucosa.

African Swine Fever

African Swine Fever is a highly contagious, highly fatal disease caused by an iridovirus distinct from the pestivirus of Classical Swine Fever. Clinical signs include high fever followed by dullness, anorexia, huddling, incoordination, dyspnoea and sometimes diarrhoea followed by death within 7–10 days in 95–100 percent of affected pigs. Once endemic, a more chronic syndrome may result with emaciation, swelling of the joints and skin ulceration. Abortion may occur in chronic forms. Lesions include severe haemorrhages throughout the carcase and bloodstained serous effusions may be found. Haemorrhages are often present on the heart, oedema is often present in the lungs and button ulcers are occasionally found in the large intestine. The lymph nodes are even more haemorrhagic than in Swine Fever.

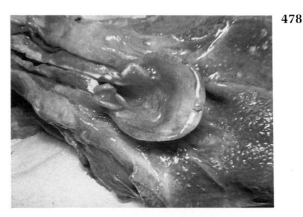

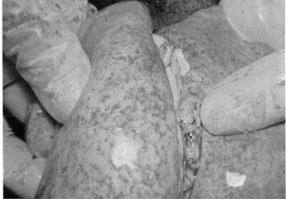

478 African Swine Fever Larynx from a case of African Swine Fever. There is oedema and congestion but no petechiae.

479 African Swine Fever Haemorrhages in the lung.

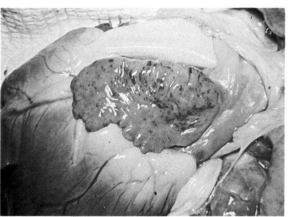

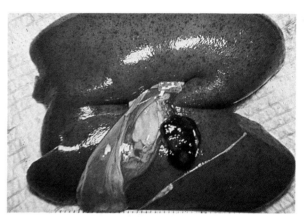

480 African Swine Fever Auricle of the heart with haemorrhages. There are no haemorrhages on the ventricular muscle in this case.

481 African Swine Fever Liver of a pig with acute African Swine Fever. Note the subcapsular haemorrhages, the distended and oedematous gall bladder and the haemorrhagic hepatic lymph node. Haemorrhage in the hepatic lymph node is one of the most consistent findings in the atypical and chronic forms of the disease.

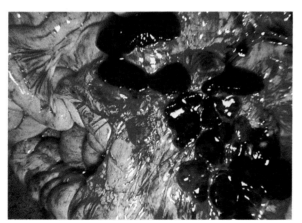

482 African Swine Fever Haemorrhagic lymph nodes may resemble blood clots. There are few, if any, other diseases in which this type of lesion can be found.

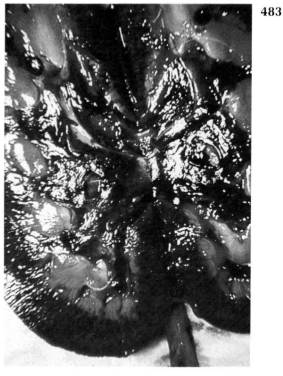

483 African Swine Fever Kidney showing severe haemorrhage into the pelvis. The petechiated 'turkey-egg' kidney of Swine Fever is less common in African Swine Fever.

Swine Vesicular Disease

Swine Vesicular disease is an infectious disease of pigs which is clinically indistinguishable from Foot and Mouth disease and is caused by an enterovirus. The virus may also cause lesions in man.

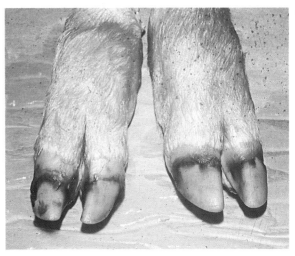

485 **Swine Vesicular Disease** Coronary band lesions, at least five days post-infection.

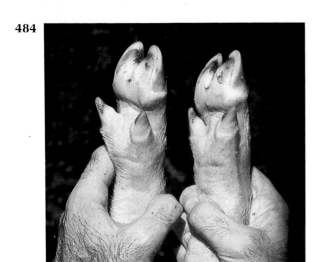

484 **Swine Vesicular Disease** Early lesions on the coronary bands, 24 hours post-infection.

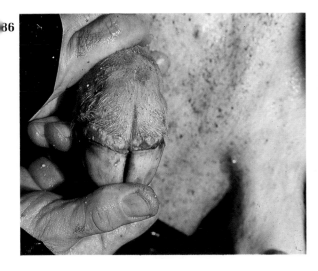

486 **Swine Vesicular Disease** Separation at the coronary band at nine days plus.

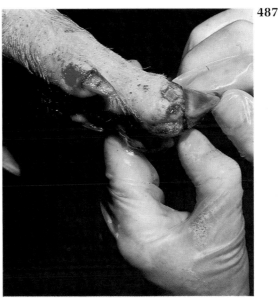

487 **Swine Vesicular Disease** Marked claw separation and a skin lesion above the supernumerary digit. Seen 13 days post-infection.

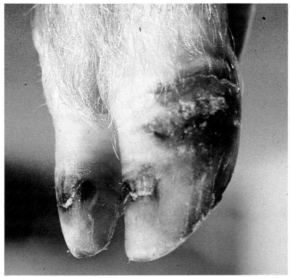

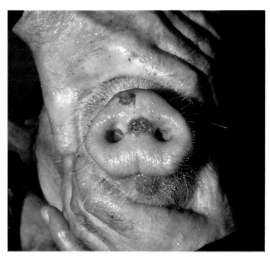

489 Swine Vesicular Disease Note the shallow ulcers on the snout and one on the lower lip.

488 Swine Vesicular Disease Late lesions with under-running of the horn in two locations on the same foot. This type of lesion appears to be caused by successive waves of infection.

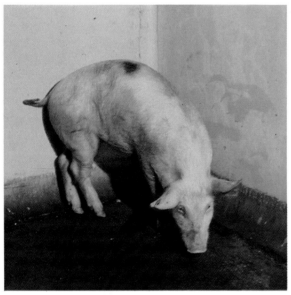

490 Foot and Mouth Disease A clinically-affected pig. Note the posture. The animal is severely lame, and would normally be lying down but has been made to stand. Affected pigs resent being disturbed.

Foot and Mouth Disease

This very contagious disease is characterised by fever (to 41°C, 106°F), the formation of vesicles on the coronary band of the foot, on the tongue and on the snout. Sudden death may occur quite commonly in sucking piglets. The initial signs are often those of severe lameness and reluctance to move. The disease affects pigs, cattle, sheep and other cloven hooved animals unlike Swine Vesicular Disease. It is difficult to distinguish between the two diseases on clinical grounds alone, and confirmation of diagnosis must be carried out by laboratory means.

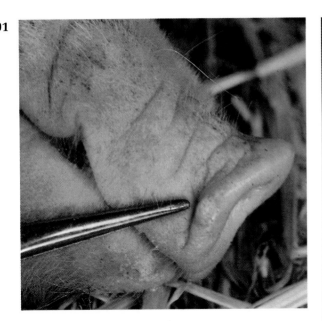

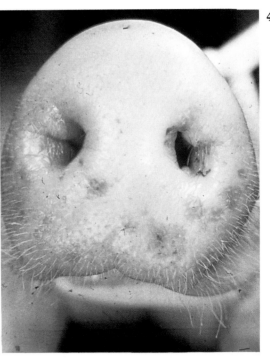

491 Foot and Mouth Disease Vesicle on the snout of a pig affected with Foot and Mouth Disease. These vesicles rupture very quickly but fluid from them is the best source of virus for diagnosis.

492 Foot and Mouth Disease An early case, the vesicles on the nose having ruptured recently leaving shallow ulcers.

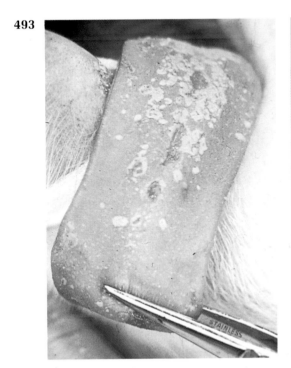

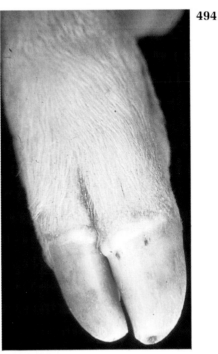

493 Foot and Mouth Disease Lesions on the tongue; ruptured and unruptured vesicles.

494 Foot and Mouth Disease Unruptured vesicles along the coronary band in an early case.

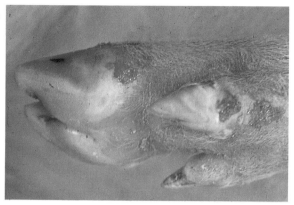

495 Foot and Mouth Disease The vesicles on the feet have ruptured recently leaving raw, shallow ulcers.

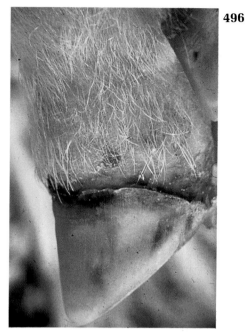

496 Foot and Mouth Disease Note the marked separation at the coronary band.

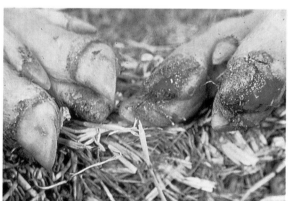

497 Foot and Mouth Disease Marked separation occurring at the coronary band and severe heel lesions.

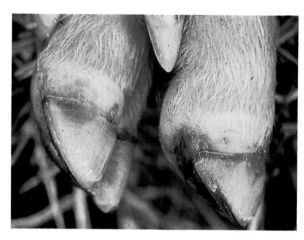

498 Foot and Mouth Disease Thimbling of the horn occurring in older lesions.

Vesicular Exanthema

This vesicular disease of pigs is caused by a calicivirus which originally came from sealions in California. It has not been seen since 1959 but might appear again at any time. The lesions and clinical signs are similar to those of Foot and Mouth Disease. Primary lesions may occur on the snout and be accompanied by fever. They then spread to the lips, tongue and coronary bands.

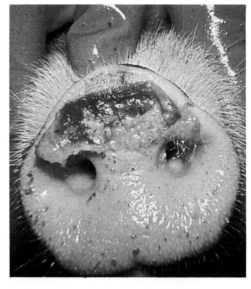

499 Vesicular Exanthema Snout of a pig with primary lesions of Vesicular Exanthema. Note the ragged area resulting from a ruptured vesicle.

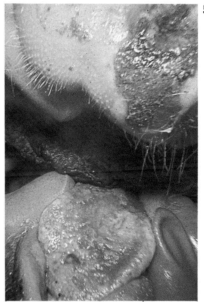

500 Vesicular Exanthema Tongue of a pig with vesicular exanthema.

Vesicular Stomatitis

This vesicular disease of pigs is difficult to distinguish from Foot and Mouth Disease on clinical grounds. It is caused by a rhabdovirus which also affects cattle and horses. Lameness is usually the most obvious clinical sign. The disease is found principally on the eastern seaboard of the United States.

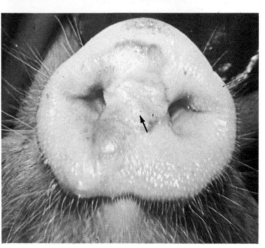

501 Vesicular Stomatitis Vesicles on the snout of a pig with Vesicular Stomatitis. Note the large blanched area (arrow).

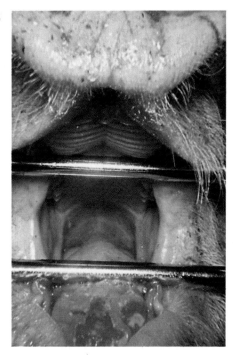

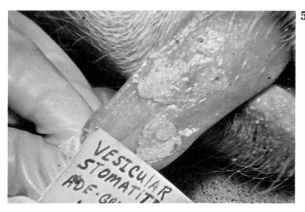

503 Vesicular Stomatitis Tongue from a case of Vesicular Stomatitis. Note the pale patches which are fibrinous exudate over the site of ruptured vesicles.

502 Vesicular Stomatitis Oral cavity of a pig with Vesicular Stomatitis. Note the freshly-ruptured vesicles on the tongue.

504

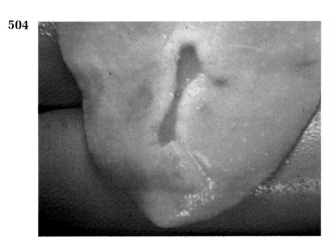

505

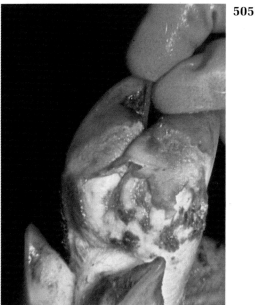

504 Vesicular Stomatitis Tongue from a case of Vesicular Stomatitis. Note the healing ulcer on the site of a vesicle.

505 Vesicular Stomatitis Foot from an early case of Vesicular Stomatitis. Note the large ruptured vesicle on the heel. The lesion has caused under-running of the newly-formed horn at the heel.

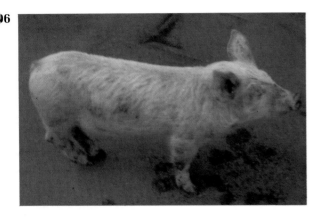

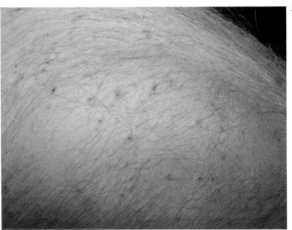

Swine Pox

An infectious disease caused by a pox virus which appears as circular, 1–3 cm lesions on the skin of the belly flanks, face and head in young pigs. The disease begins with fever after which the lesions appear as red circular papules. These develop to give a transient vesicular stage and almost immediately the vesicles burst to give a weeping lesion over which black scabs form rapidly. Affected pigs are often hairy and growth is depressed. Diagnosis is based on the presence of pox virus particles in the early lesions. The disease is mild in immune herds but can be acute in recently infected herds and then causes mortality. An important vector could be the pig louse *Haematopinus suis*.

506 Swine Pox An affected eight-week-old piglet. Note the distribution of the lesions and the length of the hair coat.

507 Swine Pox Typical lesions of Swine Pox at the papular stage. Note the red colour of the early lesions and their small size.

508 Swine Pox in a sucking piglet showing lesions in various stages of development.

509 Swine Pox Hindquarters of a coloured pig. Note the way in which the lesions are raised and are still visible. This raised nature is not so noticeable in the white pigs where colour forms the main diagnostic feature.

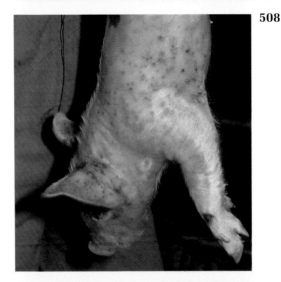

508

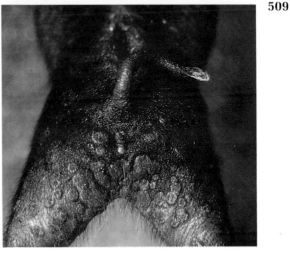

509

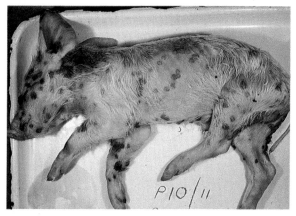

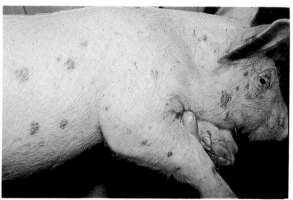

51

511 Swine Pox Scab formation in the later stages of the disease.

510 Swine Pox Carcase of a six-week-old pig which has died whilst infected with Pig Pox. Note the distribution of the lesions.

Congenital Tremor A-II

Two types of Congenital Tremor of the 'A' series are of infectious origin and the most important is A-I which is caused by congenital infection with Swine Fever. A-II occurs in a high proportion of litters and affects more than 80% of piglets in affected litters. Affected piglets are born with tremor but mortality is usually low unlike the situation in A-I. This disease is also of viral origin and occurs in the progeny of susceptible sows and affects a variable proportion of the litter. Piglets tremble while awake and may die if unable to feed. Those which die are often found to have small or underdeveloped cerebellums and histological lesions including demyelination.

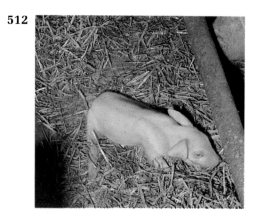

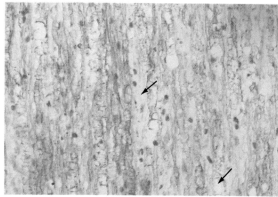

512 Congenital Tremor A-II An affected four-day-old piglet from a litter with eight trembling piglets, two normal piglets and three stillborn piglets.

513 Congenital Tremor A-II Histological section of cerebral white matter from a pig with Congenital Tremor A-II. Note the demyelination (arrows).

Diseases of Complex Aetiology

Gastro-oesophageal Ulceration

Ulceration of the pars oesophagea of the stomach is most commonly encountered in adult and finishing pigs but can occur at any age. Ulceration is preceded by parakeratosis of the stratified squamous epithelium with or without surface erosions. Initially the surface has a rough, corrugated, irregular appearance and is often a yellow-brown colour, due to an affinity for bile. In many cases erosions gradually coalesce, deepen and form deep, pitted ulcers which may envelop the whole pars oesophagea. Cessation of ulcer formation may occur, with healing, or the ulcerogenic process may continue, leading to a variety of clinical signs depending mainly on the rate of blood loss. Sudden death due to massive haemorrhage into the stomach may occur, or, at the other end of the scale, affected pigs gradually become anaemic and lose condition. In addition, clinical signs include grinding of teeth, vomition and periods of anorexia.

This is a disorder of multifactorial aetiology, but increased prevalence has been demonstrated when pigs are fed whey, finely ground diets low in fibre, or diets deficient in vitamin E or selenium.

514 Gastro-oesophageal ulcer Death in this case was due to haemorrhage from a gastro-oesophageal ulcer. Note the very pale carcase and watery blood from the incised left brachial plexus.

515 Normal pars oesophagea The scissors on the right point to the diverticulum, those on the left to the opening of the oesophagus.

516 Parakeratosis of pars oesophagea An early stage in gastro-oesophageal ulceration.

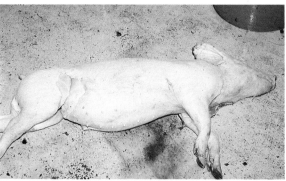

514

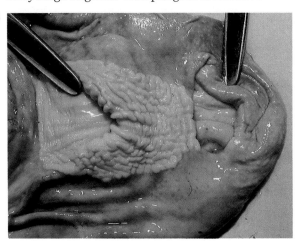

515

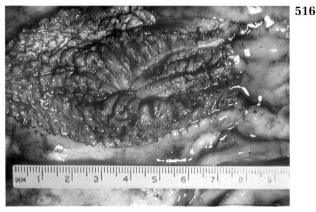

516

517

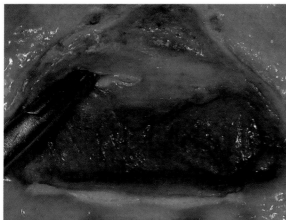

51[

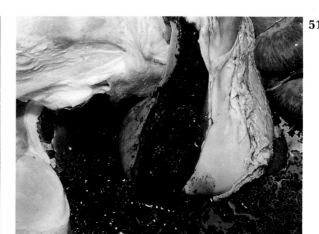

519

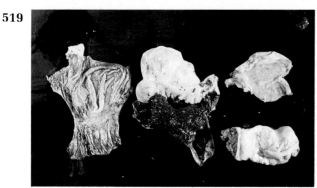

517 Gastro-oesophageal ulcer Note the crater-like erosion of the mucosa. The point of the forceps lies in the oesophageal exit.

518 Gastro-oesophageal ulcer The opened stomach of the pig from **514**. Note the large amount of clotted blood.

519 Gastro-oesophageal ulceration Death from gastric ulceration may be so rapid (as in case **514**) that altered blood may not reach the rectum or faeces. In this case it has reached the caecum (centre) but not the colon (right). Altered blood can readily be washed from the mucosa (left) in contrast to the situation in colitis.

520

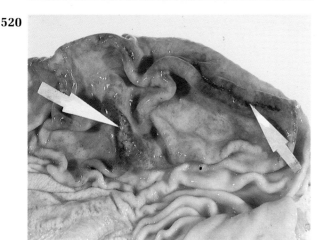

520 Gastric ulceration Ulcers in the fundus following the rugae. These lesions are often seen after weaning under stressful conditions.

52[

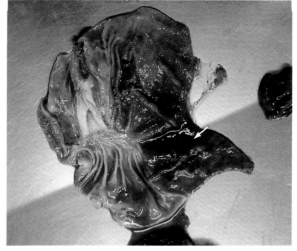

521 Gastric ulceration In many enteric conditions in which dehydration occurs, achlorhydria of the stomach is associated with congestion and haemorrhagic gastritis (arrow). Stomach from a pig with chronic swine dysentery.

Prolapse of the Uterus

Prolapse of one or both uterine horns usually occurs immediately or soon after farrowing. Occasional cases have been seen in maiden gilts after oestrus. Cases are usually sporadic but several cases may arise over a short period. Some are preceded by prolapse of the vagina and it is possible that the long muscular cervix prevents eversion of the whole womb. In the majority of cases the cause is not known but small outbreaks do occur.

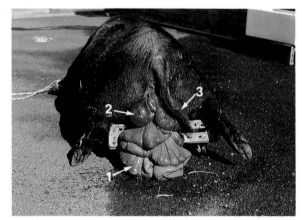

522 Prolapse of the uterus (1), bladder (2) and rectum (3) in a two-year-old sow.

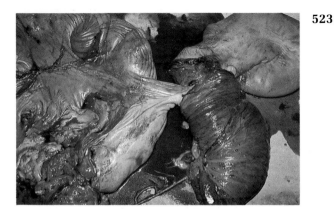

523 Uterine prolapse Dissected specimen of the uterus from a three-year-old sow post-farrowing showing invagination of the left uterine horn.

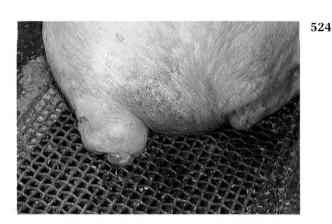

524 Vaginal cervical prolapse in a sow immediately before farrowing.

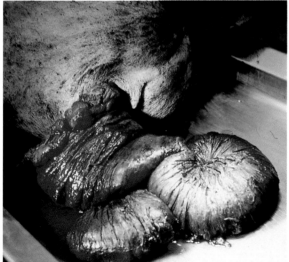

525

525 Uterine prolapse Complete prolapse of the uterus in a mature sow.

Rectal Prolapse/Rectal Stricture

In recent years prolapse of the rectal mucosa has become more common in rearing pigs within the 10 to 90 kg weight range. Certain specific conditions are known to cause prolapse *e.g.* straining from urethritis or proctitis and excessive slope in the floor of housed sows. However, in the majority of cases involving the modern hybrid, rapidly-growing pig, the cause is not clear. High gut fill, constipation, lack of fibre and other nutritional factors have been highlighted. Rectal stricture (complete or partial) frequently follows natural resolution of a damaged prolapsed rectum.

Where natural resolution of the prolapsed rectum is allowed to occur, pigs may develop complete rectal stricture while partial stricture of the rectum is commonly found when the survivors are slaughtered. In the United States, *Salmonella typhimurium* has been associated with the disease. However, cases of rectal stricture may occur sporadically without any apparent precipitating cause being detected.

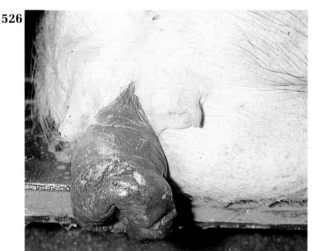

526

526 Rectal prolapse Rectal prolapse in a farrowing sow. The animal recovered after replacement of the prolapse.

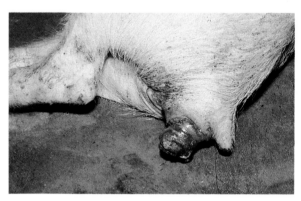

52

527 Rectal prolapse in a 16 kg weaner, two days after onset.

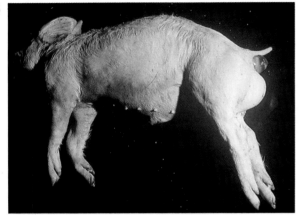

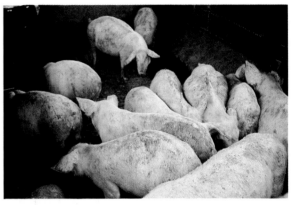

528 Rectal prolapse A six-week-old male weaner with rectal prolapse following straining after obstruction of the urethra with calculi.

529 Rectal stricture Twelve pigs with rectal stricture from a farm with a high incidence. Note the variation in bodily condition.

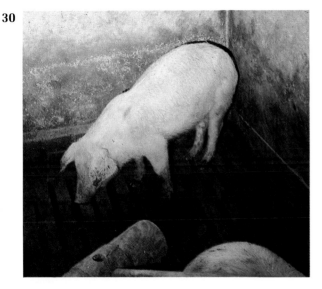

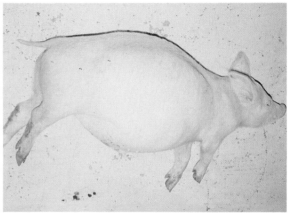

531 Rectal stricture (complete) in a 40 kg pig. Note grossly distended abdomen and loss of condition.

530 Rectal stricture Pig affected by rectal stricture adopting the typical stance. Note the distended abdomen.

532

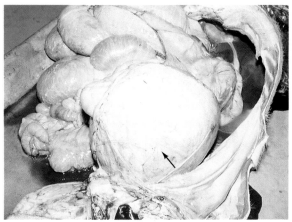

532 Rectal stricture Photograph taken after necropsy of the pig in **531**. Note the grossly distended rectum (arrow).

53

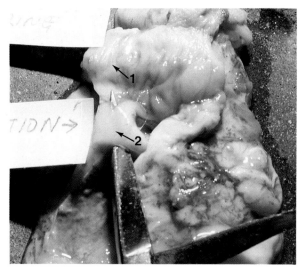

533 Rectal stricture Dissected anus and rectum from **531** showing the anal ring (1), and the fibrous constriction, through which the point of the scissors is inserted (2).

534

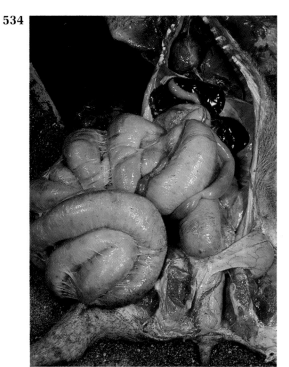

534 Rectal stricture The carcase of a pig with rectal stricture, opened to show the enlarged rectum.

535

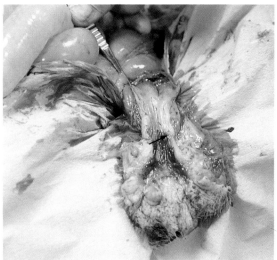

535 Rectal Stricture Rectum dissected to show inflammation and thickening at the site of stricture (arrow).

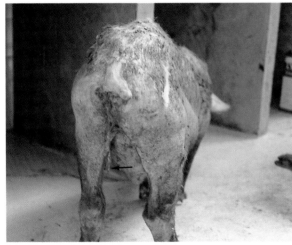

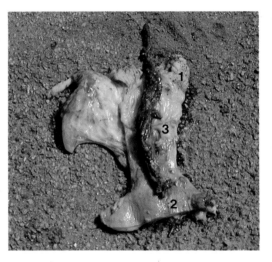

536 Rectal prolapse Rectal prolapse in a 35 kg pig, 16 days after onset. Note the remains of the damaged rectal mucosa hanging from the anus (arrow).

537 Rectal prolapse Dissected anus and rectum from the pig in **536** showing the anal ring (1), dilated thickened rectum (2), early partial stricture (3). Note the ribbon of faecal and necrotic material along the line of the lumen.

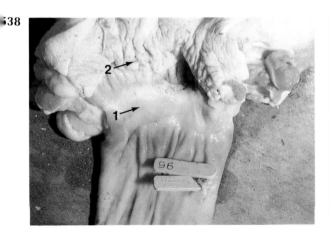

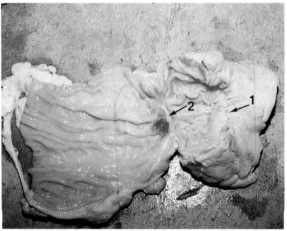

538 Partial rectal stricture Dissected anus and rectum from an 80 kg pig. This pig had survived prolapse of the rectum at 35 kg. Resolution took place naturally. Note the fibrous scar (arrow 1), and anus (arrow 2).

539 Partial rectal stricture Dissected anus (1) and rectum from an 80 kg pig. This pig survived a rectal prolapse at 31 kg liveweight. Resolution occurred naturally. The scar tissue (2) was approximately 5 cm from the anus.

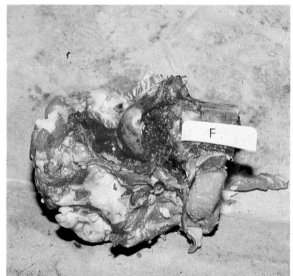

Epiphysiolysis

Separation of the head of the femur from the neck along the proximal femoral physis is termed epiphysiolysis and is more commonly found in young boars and sows. The cause is not known but several herds in which the condition was a problem have responded to increasing the calcium level in the feed (to 1%). It is also possible that the condition may be linked to osteochondrosis. Usually cases are unilateral and sudden in onset. Affected animals become paraplegic and often assume a dog sitting position: crepitus and pain may be shown on manipulation. There is no cure.

540 Epiphysiolysis Separation of the femoral head in a 10-month-old gilt. F = Femur shaft.

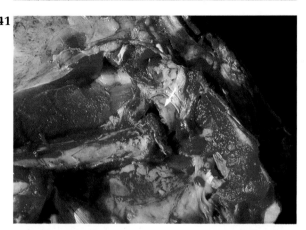

541 Epiphysiolysis Separation of femoral head (arrow) in an 80 kg finishing pig.

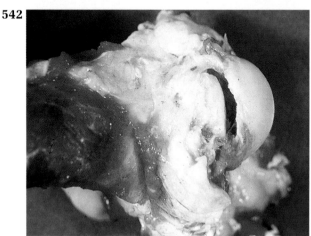

542 Epiphysiolysis Separation of the femoral head.

Apophysiolysis

Separation of the ischial tuberosity along the physeal plate is known as apophysiolysis. The condition affects both young boars and sows and may either be unilateral or bilateral. Symptoms are very similar to those of epiphysiolysis but cases have been known to repair spontaneously if left. Slippery floors may predispose to the condition.

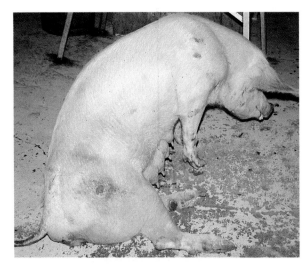

543

543 Apophysiolysis First-litter gilt in typical dog sitting position.

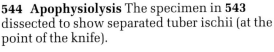

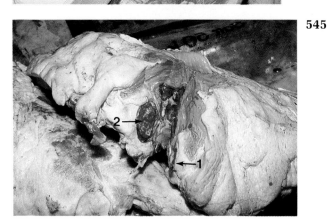

544

544 Apophysiolysis The specimen in **543** dissected to show separated tuber ischii (at the point of the knife).

545

545 Apophysiolysis Separation of the ischial tuberosity. Another view of **544** showing the ischial tuberosity (1) and tuber sacrale (2).

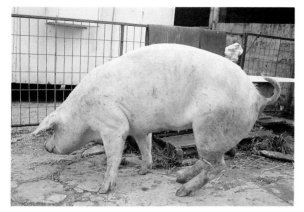

Degenerative Joint Disease/Osteochondrosis

Degenerative joint disease (DJD) is the best all-embracing term to cover Osteoarthrosis, Osteoarthritis, Polyarthritis and Arthropathy and does not imply a primary inflammatory response in either bone or cartilage. In DJD the articular epiphyseal complex is damaged, forming fissures, flaps and craters, while the primary lesion in osteochondrosis involves the articular epiphyseal growth component of the articular epiphyseal complex. Thus the latter condition may predispose to the former. Clinical signs are extremely diverse according to the nature and severity of lesions and the number of joints involved. The severity of lesions may not always be associated with the severity of clinical signs.

546 Degenerative joint disease A 14-month-old gilt with degenerative joint disease of both stifle joints. Note the posture.

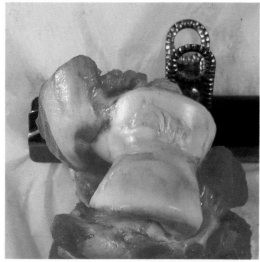

547 Degenerative joint disease The humeral condyles of a 120 kg gilt. Note the ridging of the articular cartilage.

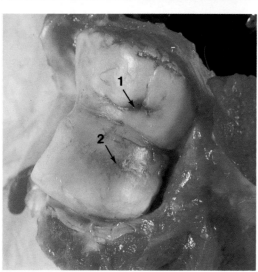

548 Degenerative joint disease The humeral condyles of an 80 kg pig. Note the fissure (1) and thinning of cartilage (2).

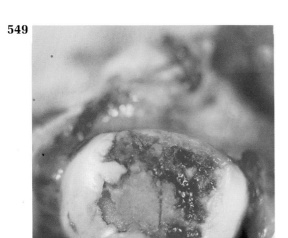

549 Degenerative joint disease Femoral head of a 120 kg gilt, showing erosion of the articular cartilage exposing underlying bone.

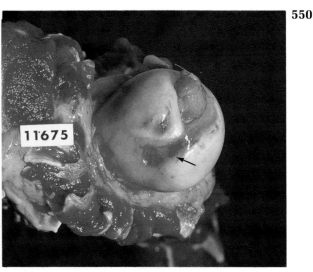

550 Degenerative joint disease Note the erosion of articular cartilage (arrow).

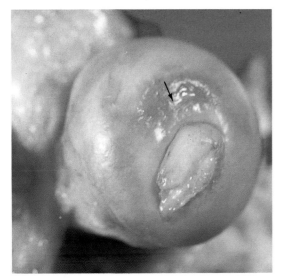

551 Degenerative joint disease Head of femur. Note erosion of the articular cartilage (arrow).

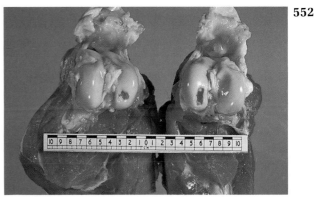

552 Degenerative joint disease Bilateral osteochondrosis of mesial condyles of the femur.

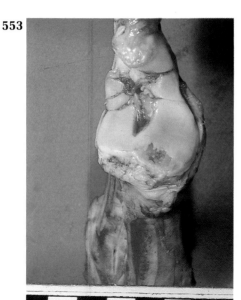

553 Degenerative joint disease Osteochondrosis of the radius.

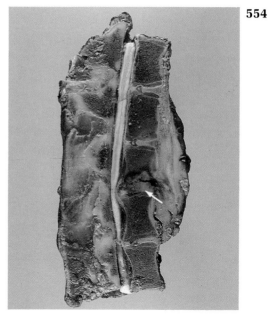

554 Degenerative joint disease Degenerative disc lesion (arrow) in a 40 kg weaner. The pressure on the spinal cord caused posterior paralysis.

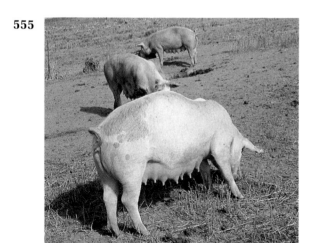

555 Humpy back (Kyphosis) A sow from an affected herd. This animal is clinically normal. Humpy back in sows is most obvious when body condition is low. The aetiology is obscure.

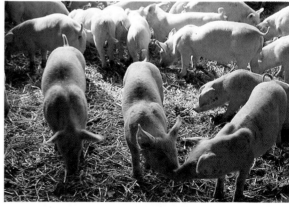

556 Humpy back A group of 10-week-old growers from the same herd as the sows shown in **555**. Some severely affected animals fail to grow and die, sometimes suddenly.

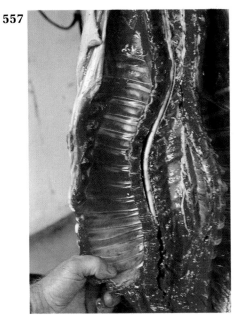

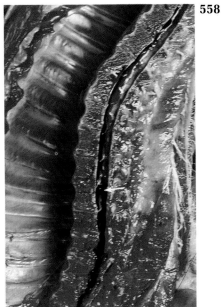

557 Humpy back Spinal curvature is pronounced in this grower from the group shown in **556**. The spinal canal widens at the peak of the curve and narrows in the trough.

558 Humpy back In badly affected pigs fighting or other movements may result in the rupture of spinal arteries and death from spinal cord compression. Note the blood clot in the vertebral canal (arrow).

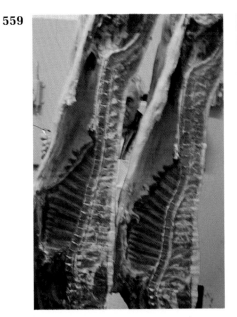

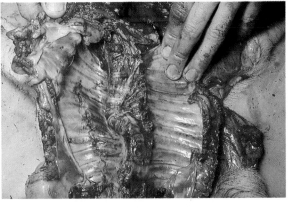

560 Congenital kinky back in a suckling piglet.

559 Humpy back In some cases the hump is postural. Here two humpy back pigs from the same herd have been sawn in two at slaughter. In one (left) the spine has straightened; in the other, the spinal curvature has remained and skeletal changes are present.

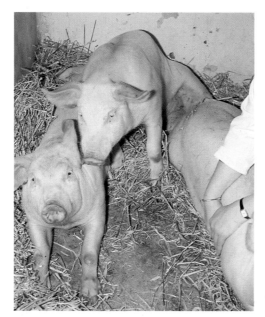

Electrocution

Electrocution occurs on the farm from time to time. Pigs are particularly susceptible because of their inquisitive behaviour and moist snouts. Death may occur immediately, or more commonly they may be found alive with paralysis due to fracture of a spinal vertebra or long bone. This is caused by massive spasm of the muscle in one area. Fractures of the spine and femur may occur during stunning and slaughter with the use of electrodes, especially if the equipment or technique is faulty.

561 Electrocution Three 40 kg weaners unable to move because of posterior paralysis – a sequel to on-farm electrocution via the food trough.

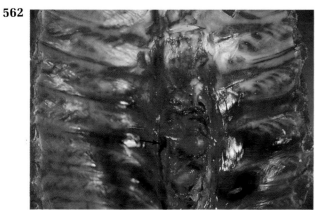

562 Electrocution Lumbar area from a pig in **561** – Note the spinal fracture (arrow).

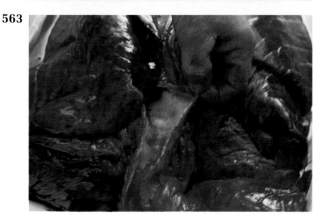

563 Electrocution Lungs from an electrocuted sow with trachea opened to show agonal froth.

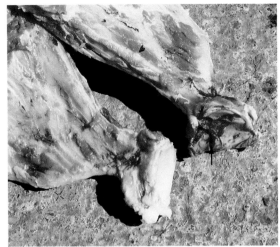

564 Electrocution Scapula from an electrocuted finisher (left) with fractures (arrow) of the joint surface caused by muscular contraction. A control scapula is shown on the right.

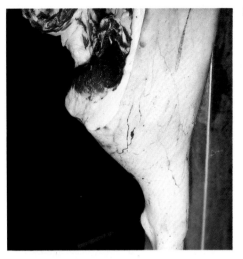

565 Electrocution Haemorrhage into the hind limb muscles. This was due to faulty electrical stunning.

Deviation of the Lower Jaw (Mandibular Malalignment)

This condition is commonly seen in sows and boars usually confined in stalls or by tethers. In some herds the deviation may be to one side only, if for example, sows are tethered allowing one-way movement of the head towards food and water. Two forms of Mandibular Malalignment have been described.

In type A the convexity of the normal condylar articular surface of the mandible is lost along with loss of curvature along both the longitudinal and transverse axis. In type B the convexity of the condyles is relatively normal but there is a significant reduction in the height of the vertical ramus on one side to which side the mandible is also deviated. This condition should not be confused with atrophic rhinitis.

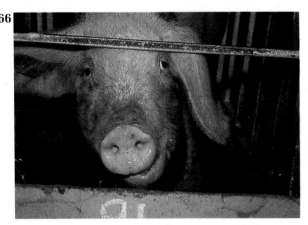

566 Deviation of the lower jaw (Mandibular malalignment). Jaw deviated to the left.

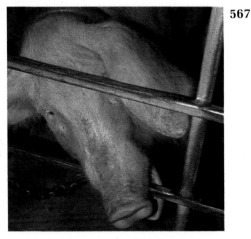

567 Deviation of the lower jaw (Mandibular malalignment). The same animal as shown in **566**. This sow continually chewed the bar to her left.

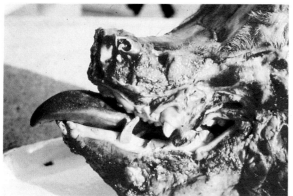

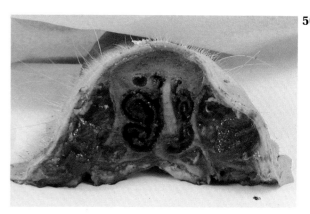

568 Brachygnathia superior Shortening of the upper jaw in an adult Large White boar. There was no evidence of atrophic rhinitis when the snout was cut transversely between premolars one and two.

569 Septal defect The snout of a 70 kg pig with twisting of the snout. This was not a case of atrophic rhinitis. Note the deviation of the medial septum leaving normal turbinates in an enlarged space on the left side while causing pressure and distortion of the turbinates on the right.

Haemorrhagic Disease

Haemorrhagic disorders may be due to well-known poisons such as rodenticides (*e.g.* warfarin) but in other cases the cause may not be determined. Mycotoxins may also cause haemorrhagic diathesis. Minor outbreaks have been seen in sows after farrowing.

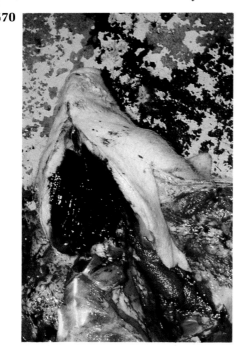

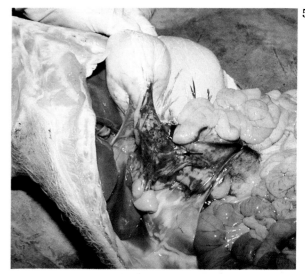

571 Haemorrhagic disease in a 45 kg pig. This was a feed-induced disorder of unknown aetiology. Haemorrhagic pancreatitis was a special feature of this particular case (arrow).

570 Haemorrhagic disease in a 45 kg pig. This was a feed-induced disorder of unknown aetiology. Note the submandibular haemorrhage.

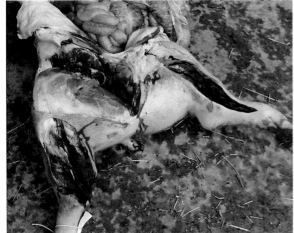

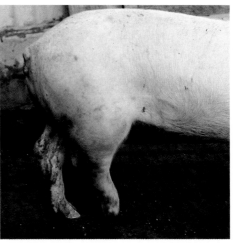

572 Haemorrhagic disease The same animal as shown in **571**. Note its severe bilateral subcutaneous haemorrhage.

573 Haemorrhagic disease Note the swelling of the right stifle joint, lameness and evidence of blood trickling down inside the right hind leg from the anus. This animal was fed stale bread and mycotoxicosis was suspected. The condition responded to vitamin K therapy.

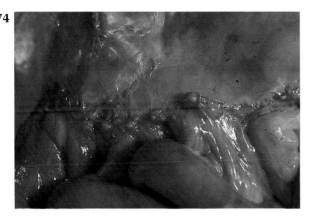

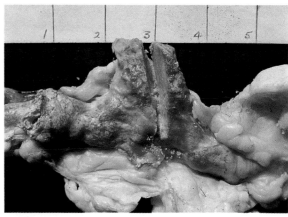

574 Osseous metaplasia in a four-year-old sow. Note the spicules of bone in the mesentery of the small intestines. These bones may be so sharp that it is possible they may tear the mesentery and stimulate torsions.

575 Osseous metaplasia Bone in perirenal fat. Age unknown.

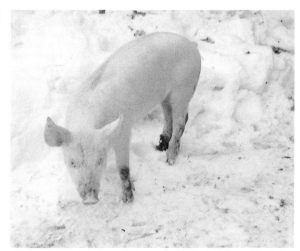

Gangrene

Gangrenous lesions of the extremities, especially of the ears, may occur as part of other systemic infections, notably those of a toxic nature. Apart from these, the effects of frostbite and ergot poisoning, gangrene is rare.

576 Gangrene A 17 kg weaner with gangrene of the right hind lower leg. Cause unknown. Note that the animal is bearing weight on the foot. Several pigs in this group were affected but in each case only one hind leg was involved.

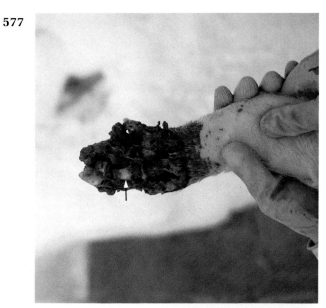

577 Gangrene A close-up of the lower right hind leg of the pig in **576.** Note the exposure of metatarsal bone (arrow).

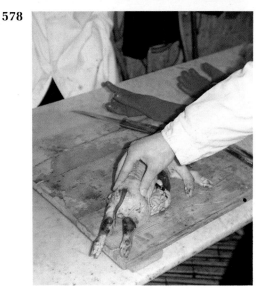

578 Wet gangrene of the tail and both hocks.

Transit Erythema

Transit erythema, also known as lime burning or urine scalding usually occurs during transit or while holding in pens without bedding for an undue length of time prior to slaughter. Skin contact with faeces, urine, lime or various disinfectants are the most common causes. The lesions are indistinct until the affected animals pass through the scalding tank. Lesions vary from distinct multifocal, pale pink or dark red areas, to more severe, confluent blemishes of the skin which vary greatly in severity. Some cases fade as the carcase sets, while others will require localised trimming or even skinning of the whole carcase.

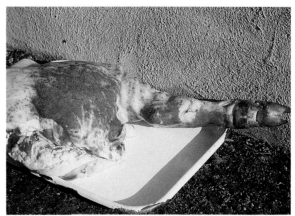

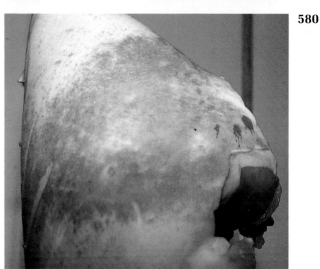

579 Transit erythema A ham from an 80 kg pig after slaughter, plotting and dehairing by hot flame.

580 Transit erythema A ham from of an 80 kg pig after slaughter, plotting and dehairing by machine.

581 Transit erythema The belly of an 90 kg pig after slaughter, plotting and dehairing by machine.

582 Transit erythema Severe case.

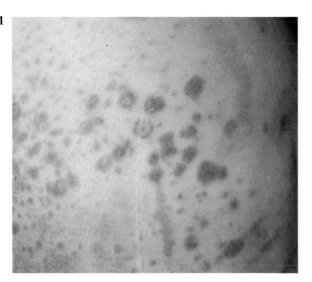

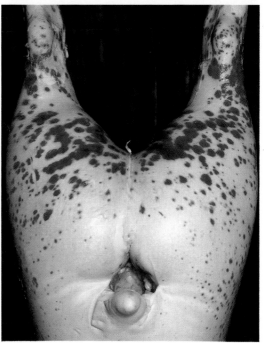

583

584

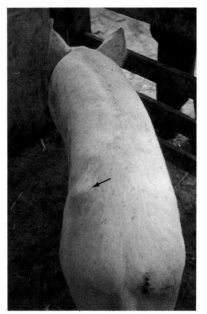

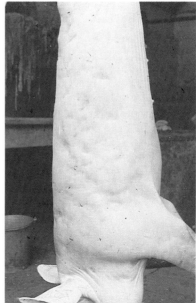

583 Skin-dimpling (arrow) The cause of this condition is not known. However it is congenital.

584 Skin-dimpling Multifocal lesions at slaughter (uncertain aetiology).

585

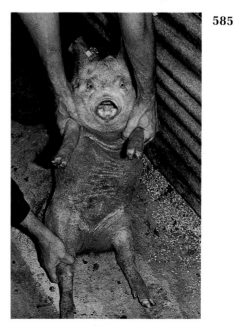

585 Dermatitis Severe contact dermatitis due to chloride of lime dusted onto a wet floor and not washed off.

586 Photosensitisation Both ears are badly affected.

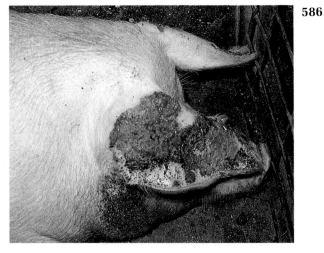

587 Photosensitisation Udder lesions in a sow.

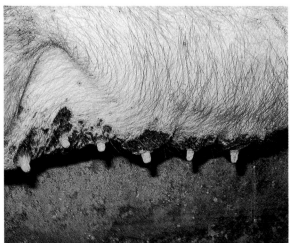

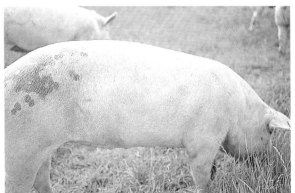

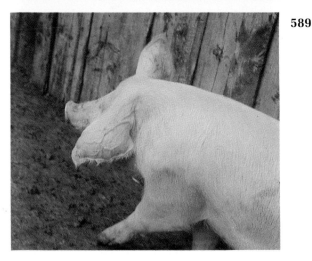

588 Sunburn Although this was a mild case this gilt had typical nervous signs.

589 Aural haematoma in 70 kg finishing pig. Note the swelling of the left ear. This condition frequently results from the head shaking associated with sarcoptic mange. Resolution of the lesion results in a 'cauliflower ear'.

Stillbirths

Stillbirths refer to foetuses born dead at full term and fall into two categories, prepartum death – Type 1 and intrapartum death – Type II. The former are less common and can be distinguished from the latter by the degree of autolysis present and the absence of other features found in Type II stillbirths. The latter occur because of anoxia during the birth process for different reasons, *e.g.* premature rupture of the cord, premature separation of the placenta, knotted cord, twisting of the cord, haematoma of the cord and more specifically carbon monoxide poisoning. Prolonged birth interval is also a significant factor and more Type II stillbirths occur in the last third of parturition.

Anoxia during birth causes increased peristalsis of the lower gut, leading to excretion of meconium and the initiation of breathing, resulting in the inhalation of mucus and meconium pellets into the trachea and larger bronchi. In addition the lungs will be un-expanded (atelectatic) and the chest cavity full of straw-coloured fluid. However, in some cases severely anoxic piglets are born alive with incomplete lung inflation (partial atelectasis). They are extremely weak and cannot compete for a teat and die fairly soon after birth.

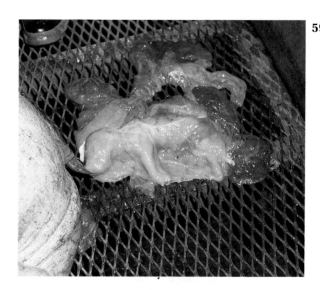

590 Stillbirth Type II In this case the piglet is still enveloped in placental membrane.

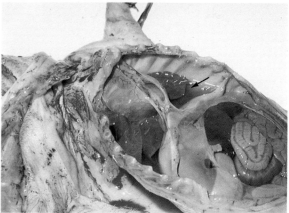

591 Stillbirth Type II The piglet from **590**. Note the excessive straw-coloured fluid in the chest cavity (arrow) and atelectatic lungs.

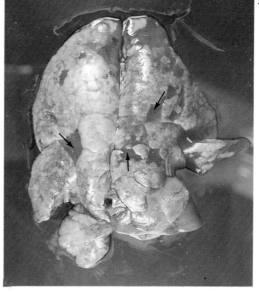

592 Stillbirth Type II Lungs from a newborn piglet with partial atelectasis (arrows).

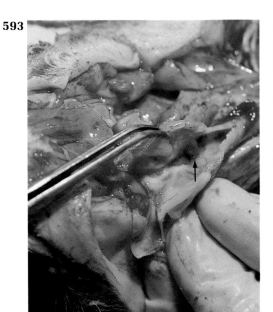

593

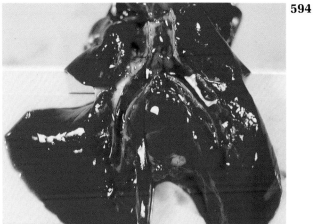

594

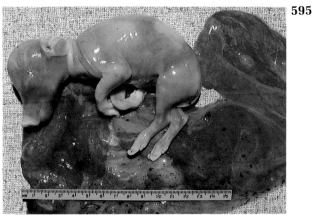

595

593 Stillbirth Type II The piglet from **590**. The trachea has been incised to expose pellets of meconium (arrow).

594 Stillbirth Type II A lung from a type II stillborn piglet showing a plug of meconium at the bifurcation of the trachea.

595 Stillbirth Type II Retarded foetal development in one piglet in a litter due to twisting of the umbilical cord twice round the neck.

596 Stillbirth Type II Retarded foetal development due to twisting of the umbilical cord round the neck and abdomen.

597 Stillbirth Type II The same piglet with the umbilical cord unwound.

596

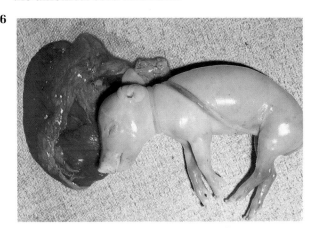

597

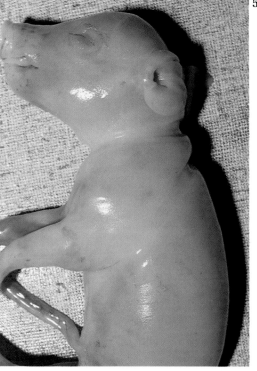

598

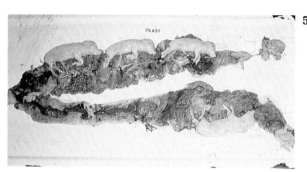

599 Stillbirth Type I Foetal death due to ascending uterine infection. Cause unknown.

598 Uterine rupture during farrowing The knife points to a tear in the uterus. Note the decomposing emphysematous foetus.

Torsion of the Gut

The pig is particularly susceptible to torsion of various parts of the digestive tract. One of the most common, torsion of the mesentery (bloody gut, red gut, whey bloat), is often mistakenly diagnosed as haemorrhagic enteritis. The whole of the small bowel and large bowel rotates around the root of the mesentery and is more frequently encountered when pigs are fed skimmed milk or whey. The cause is unknown but may be preceded by a fermentation in the large bowel, allowing the caecum to act as a lever on the rest of the gut, but this is only conjecture. Torsions have been

reported in pigs following general anaesthesia. Pigs die suddenly and, if seen before death, show signs of severe pain.

Sows fed once daily are more likely to suffer a torsion of the stomach and spleen as opposed to sows fed twice daily. An association with *Clostridium* novyi infection (**283** and **284**) has been suggested. In all cases of torsion, decomposition of the carcase is rapid. Various torsions are depicted in the following photographs.

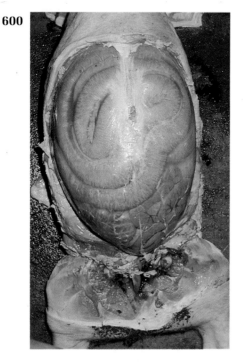

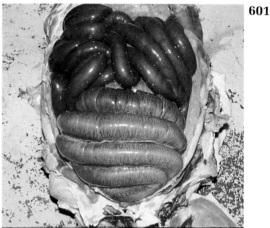

600 Distension of the gut Distension of the large intestine with the peritoneal membrane still intact. This distension will cause death due to shock, without a torsion necessarily occurring.

601 Torsion of the mesentery in a 65 kg pig. Note the position of the large intestine.

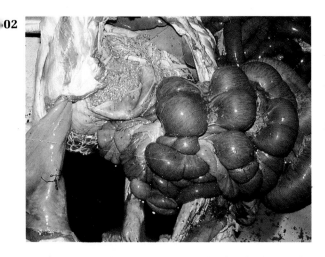

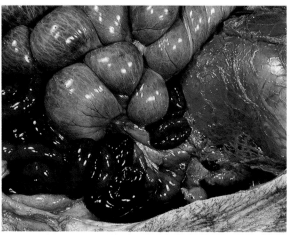

602 Torsion of the mesentery The pig from **601** with the gut removed. Note the excess blood-stained fluid and full stomach.

603 Torsion of small intestines only in a 65 kg pig.

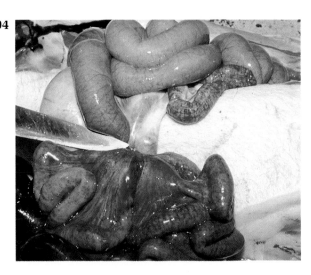

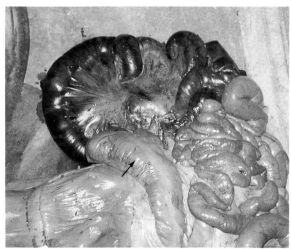

604 Torsion of a loop of the small intestine The knife points to the point of torsion. Note the acutely congested (almost necrotic) loops of small intestine.

605 Torsion of the terminal ileum Note the normal caecum (arrow).

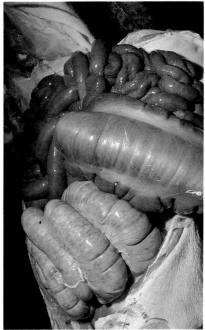

607 Torsion of the large intestine and caecum
Note the normal small intestines (arrow).

606 Torsion of the small intestine and caecum
in a 70 kg pig. Note the normal large intestine.

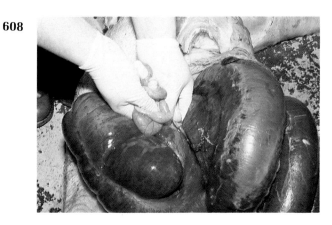

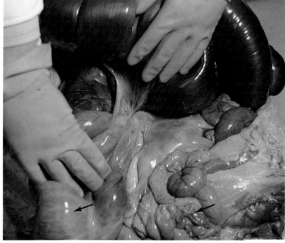

608 Torsion of the large intestine and caecum
Another view of **607**. Normal small intestines
in hand.

609 Torsion of the large intestine only Note
the normal caecum and small intestines
(arrows).

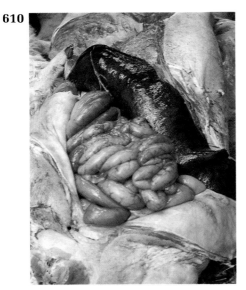

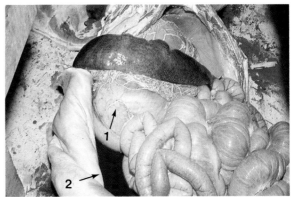

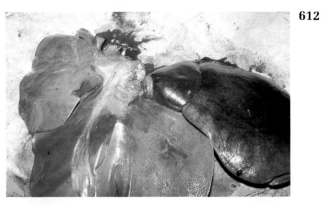

610 Torsion of the spleen in a 45 kg pig. Note the extremely enlarged, engorged spleen.

611 Torsion of Stomach and Spleen Note the enlarged, friable, engorged spleen, dilated stomach (1) and blood-stained fluid in the abdomen (2).

612 Torsion of left lobe of the liver This caused the sudden death of a five-year-old sow.

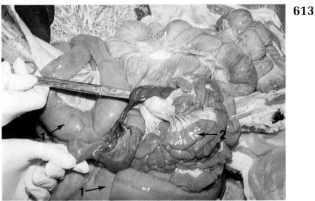

613 Intussusception of the small intestine in a 25 kg weaner. Note the dilated small intestine (1) anterior to the obstruction, and the relatively normal small intestine (2) posterior to the lesion.

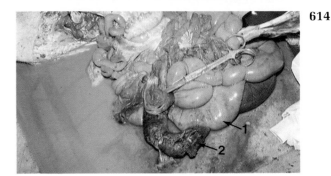

614 Intussusception Note the distension of the bowel (1) anterior to the obstruction. Arrow 2 points to the necrotic bowel.

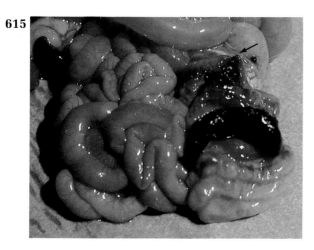

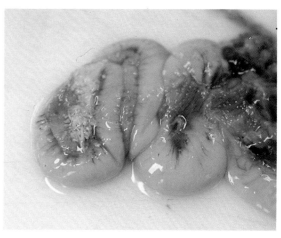

615 Impaction of large intestine with shavings in a five-day-old piglet. Note the volcano-like protrusion in the large bowel due to a sharp wood fragment almost causing penetration (arrow).

616 Sawdust Impaction The colon from a five-day-old piglet with sawdust blockage in mid colon.

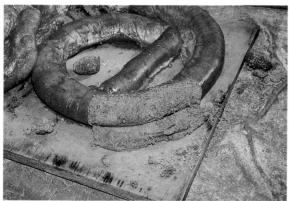

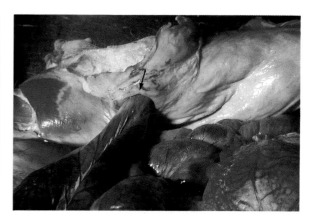

617 Impaction of the terminal ileum with sawdust The ileum from a three-year-old boar bedded on sawdust. Pigs may be bedded on sawdust without any problems arising. However, for reasons unknown, certain individuals may suddenly consume large amounts.

618 Occlusion of the small intestine due to incarceration in an umbilical hernia (arrow). Note acute congestion and dilation of the small intestine (*see* **49–51**).

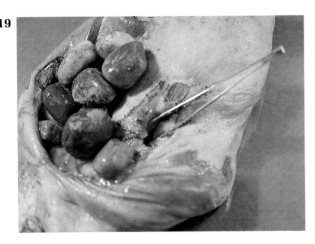

619 Stones found in the stomach of a four-year-old sow. The forceps lie in the oesophageal exit.

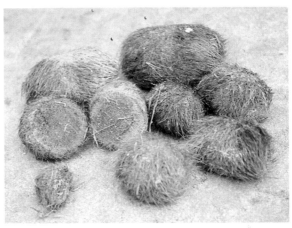

620 Hairballs A collection found in the stomachs of a group of boars kept without bedding.

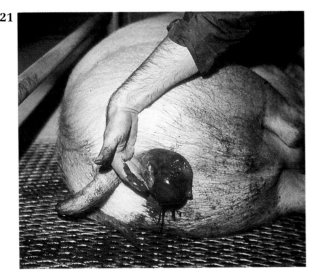

621 Vulval haematomata are common in gilts. They organise and heal rapidly if not traumatised further.

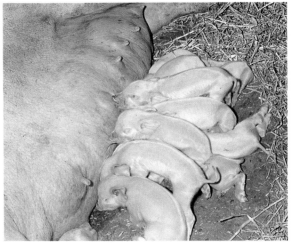

622 'Hard Udder' This condition occurs after farrowing and is associated with agalactia. Mastitis may not be present. In this picture the piglets are depressed and the hard, overfilled mammary glands are clearly visible.

173

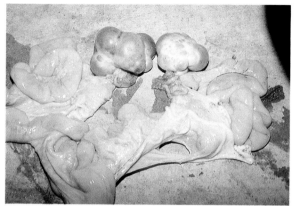

Ovarian Cysts

These occur more commonly in sows than gilts and may either be cystic corpora lutea or cystic follicles. Either may exist in the pregnant animal but are more commonly found in infertile animals. Apart from exogenous source of oestrogens and the misuse of fertility drugs, the cause is often not known.

623 Cystic ovaries in a first-litter gilt.

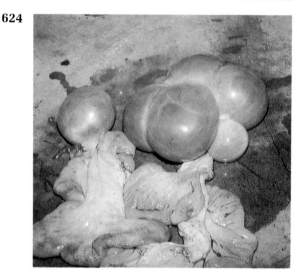

624 Cystic ovaries in a third-parity sow.

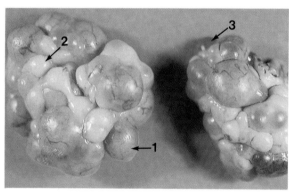

625 Normal ovaries showing a Corpus luteum (arrow 1), Corpus albicans (arrow 2), Developing Graffian follicle (arrow 3).

Navel Bleeding

Bleeding from the navel cord of neonates has been recognised in most pig-rearing countries of the world. The prevalence varies greatly from herd to herd. The whole litter may be affected but more commonly only one to three piglets in a litter develop the disorder. Affected piglets have large fleshy navels and the haemorrhage may be severe enough to kill the piglet rapidly, while in other cases piglets survive but are obviously pale and weak. There is no clotting defect in the blood and failure of the cord closure mechanism is the most likely explanation.

In one published experimental study, wood shavings used for bedding in the farrowing pen were shown to contain the causal factor. In another incident a large number of cases were noted in three herds (belonging to the same owner) with a complex nutritional problem including riboflavin deficiency. Vitamin C therapy has been recommended but it has failed to prevent the problem occurring in several trials.

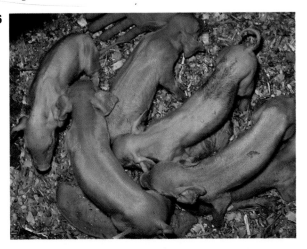

626 Navel bleeding Pale piglets associated with navel bleeding. Note the shavings being used for bedding.

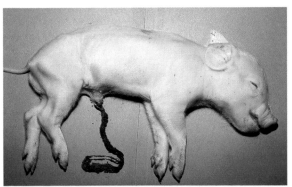

627 Navel bleeding Note the pale carcase and large fleshy navel.

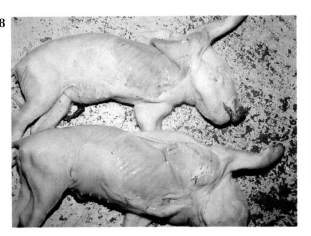

628 Navel bleeding Note the pale carcases and almost total absence of blood in the brachial plexus.

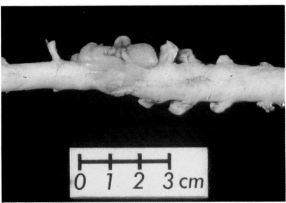

629 Neurofibrosarcoma – spinal cord This rare tumour caused compression of the spinal cord in a five-month-old pig, resulting in posterior paralysis.

630

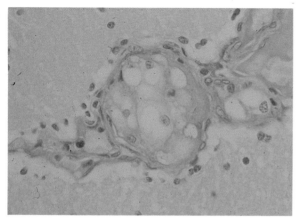

630 Fibrocartilaginous embolism of the cerebellum Two fibrocartilaginous masses, each containing cells resembling chondrocytes, are lodged in the meningeal blood vessels (Alcian blue stain). The origin of the embolus is most probably the nucleus pulposus of an intervertebral disc.

63

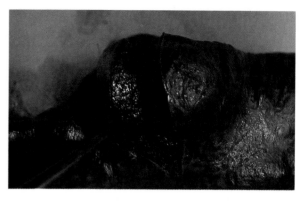

631 Haematoma of the spleen (incised) found during routine post mortem.

632

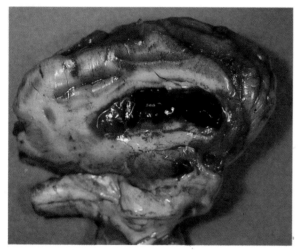

632 Brain The mid-section of the brain from a 16 kg pig. Spontaneous haemorrhage into the lateral ventricle caused the death of this pig.

63

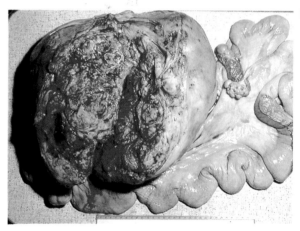

633 Ovarian/uterine tumour (leiomyoma).

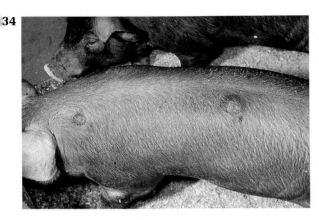

34

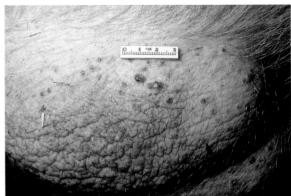

635

634 Melanomata in a Duroc These may be hereditary.

635 Multiple scrotal haemangioma

636–641 Injuries to the penis

636 The free end of the boar penis at rest, covered by the penile integument; this part of the penis is most commonly involved in injuries. Note the spiral arrangement of the tip.

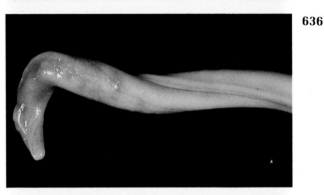

636

637 Abrasion and laceration of the penile integument and tunica albuginea, 5 cm from the penile tip. The cavernous bodies were not involved in this injury.

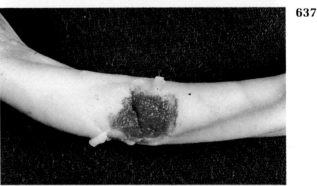

637

638 Abrasion and laceration penetrating the corpus cavernosum approximately 8 cm distal to the preputial reflection.

639 In this case the free end of the penis is severely damaged; the laceration involves both carvernous bodies and the urethra.

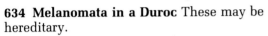

38

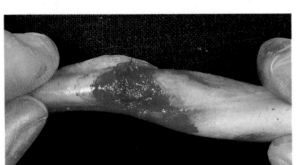

639

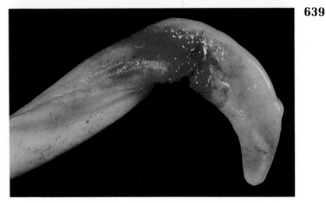

640

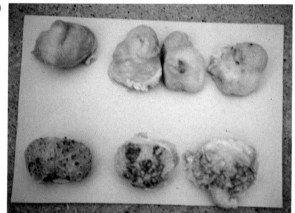

640 Preputial Ulcers The cause, and the effect of these ulcers is not known.

641

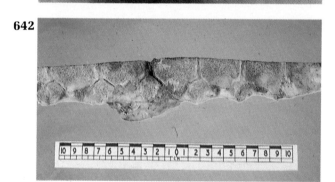

641 Spondylosis X-ray of the lumbar spine of a boar with spondylosis.

642

642 Spondylosis The same case as **641** at post mortem.

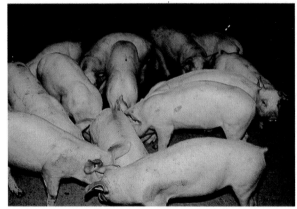

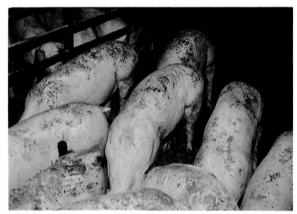

643 & 644 Colitis (grower scour) of unknown
aetiology. Morbidity may be high but there is
no mortality. Affected pigs are always dirty
(**644**). Pelleted feeds are usually involved.
When the same feed is presented as a meal the
condition resolves spontaneously (*see* **643**).

645   Colon from a pig with colitis In this case
secondary bacterial infection caused lesions
which could be confused with those of swine
dysentery (see **407-411**).

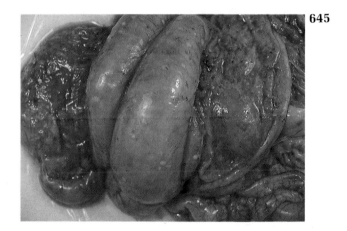

Behavioural Problems and Vices

Abnormal patterns of behaviour may develop into vices such as ear-biting, tail-biting, flank-biting and vulva biting. These vices are good examples of disorders of multifactorial or complex aetiology *i.e.* it usually requires a number of factors acting together, or in sequence, to induce a vice which may be only expressed by one individual in a group but often ultimately involves several pigs in the group.

A large number of factors have been identified and can be grouped under the main headings of social, physical and climatic environment. Examples are overstocking (liveweight kg/m²),

large group size, lack of trough space and wide variation in temperature. With tail-biting the male is more commonly bitten than the female and boars more than castrates. The initial precipitating factor may no longer be apparent by the time a specific vice becomes clinically apparent. Some of the more serious outbreaks of ear and flank biting have been noted in docked pigs in straw-based systems.

True cannibalism has been detected in outside farrowing systems. This occurs when a sow has developed the vice of killing and eating piglets belonging to other sows.

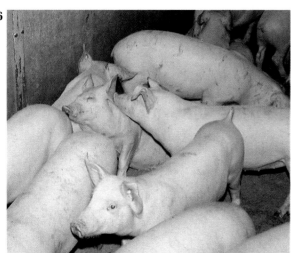

646 Ear sucking – a prelude to ear biting? Note the apparent acceptance by the pig receiving the attention.

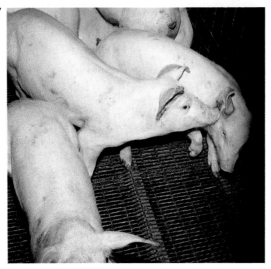

647 Ear biting Weaner actively ear-biting in a flat-deck weaner unit. In this case the ventilation system had practically failed and in addition, many weaners were suffering from sub-clinical Porcine Intestinal Adenomatosis (PIA).

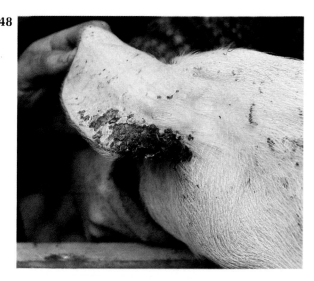

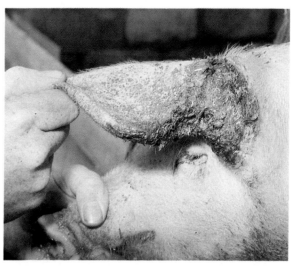

648 Ear biting Note the lesion at the base of the ear in this four-week-old piglet in a multi-suckling group.

649 Ear biting Note that there is partial healing but with evidence of breakdown due to recent attacks from pen mates.

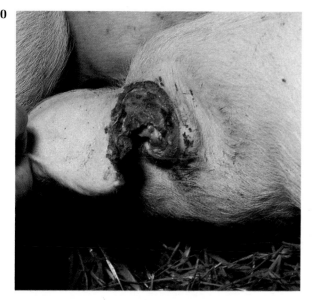

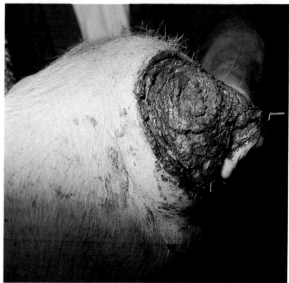

650 Ear biting An extensive wound in 14-week-old weaner on deep straw.

651 Ear biting Note the extensive scar tissue. This pig was in a group of 65 animals on straw where ear biting had been an on-going problem for 10 days.

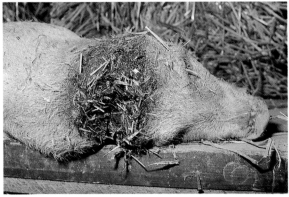

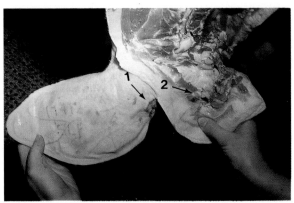

652 Ear biting Complete absence of ears – a sequel to ear biting – in a 14-week-old weaner on deep straw. The damage was caused during a 72-hour-period.

653 Ear biting This plate shows ear biting at the junction of the ear with the face (1). The green dye from ear marking has been transferred to the parotid lymph node (2). This node is the body's first line of defence to infection from ear-biting.

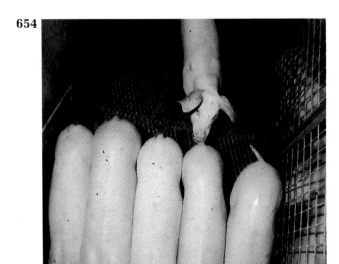

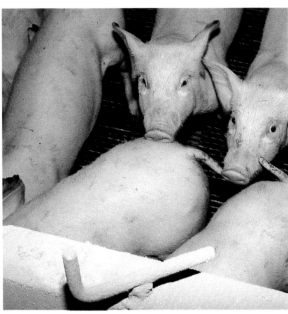

654 Tail biting The culprit caught in the act – probably frustrated because of lack of trough space. Note the bitten tails of the three pigs to the left.

655 Tail biting Two frustrated weaners attacking a pig at trough in front. Note the necrosis of the ear tips in the middle pig, also due to ear biting.

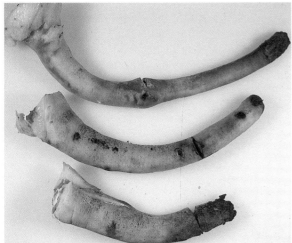

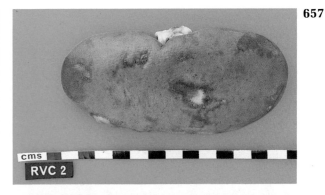

656 Bitten tails Note the abscesses – a common source of pyaemia (*see* **657**).

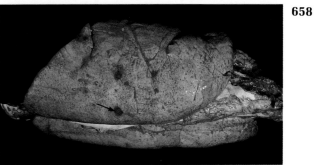

657 Pyaemic abscesses in the kidney A sequel to tail-biting.

658 Tail biting Pyaemia resulting in lung abscesses. Note the haemorrhagic zone around one abscess (arrow).

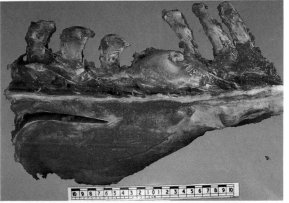

659 Tail biting Osteomyelitis of the first lumbar vertebra due to pyaemia following tail-biting. A common site.

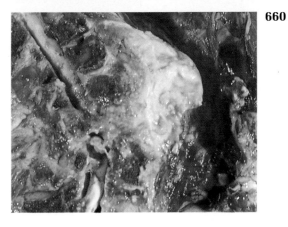

660 Tail biting Osteomyelitis of the vertebrae of the thoracic inlet due to pyaemia from tail biting. An uncommon site. See also *Actinomyces (C.) pyogenes* (**299–301**).

661

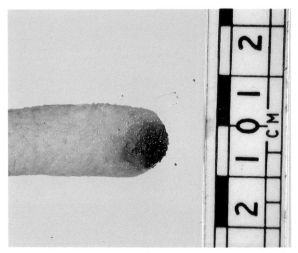

661 Tail-tip necrosis, probably the result of poor circulation following trauma to the tail tip. It has been suggested that these lesions precipitate tail-biting. They do not.

662

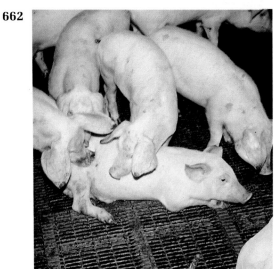

Flank Biting

Flank biting usually occurs in pigs of 14–40 kg. The disorder has been noted in pigs with and without bedding. It is usually caused by either nosing, licking and/or rubbing of one pig on another. The area selected for initial nuzzling varies widely from one pig to another – hence the diversity of lesion site depicted in these pictures. Usually the lesion occurs over the rib cage or abdomen.

662 Flank nuzzling – a prelude to flank biting Notice the apparent acceptance by the pig receiving the attention. In this case the pig on the left rubbed the recumbent pig 122 times before the latter objected. Note also the ear-biting lesions on the tip of the ear in the pig on the left.

663

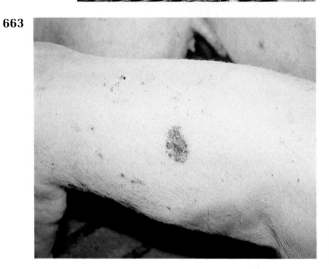

663 Flank biting lesion in a 35 kg weaner. Note the scar tissue recently rubbed off by a pen-mate.

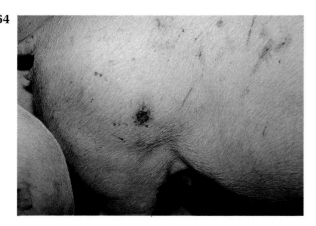

664 Flank biting In this case the lesion is on the mid-upper right leg.

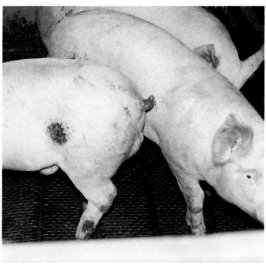

665 Flank biting in growers These pigs are housed on a punched metal floor and skin abrasions are occurring elsewhere.

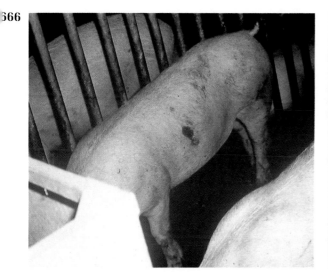

666 Healing flank biting lesion In this case the weight of pigs per square metre had exceeded the recommended figures (0.4m²/40 kg liveweight).

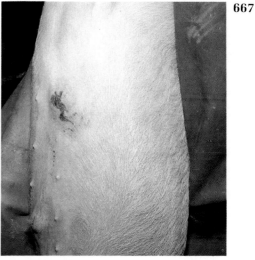

667 Nipple sucking lesion in a seven-week-old pig from flat-deck accommodation. This is not common and in this case the cause was not discovered although the culprit was.

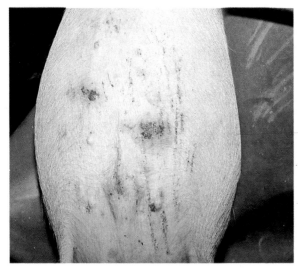

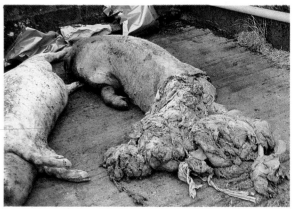

669 Pseudo-cannibalism As opposed to true cannibalism when sows will kill and eat normal piglets, pseudo-cannibalism is common if dead pigs are left in a pen for more than four hours.

668 Nipple Sucking lesion Damage to two teats. An eight-week-old weaner from flat-deck accommodation. Pen mate to the pig in **667**.

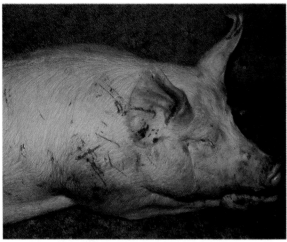

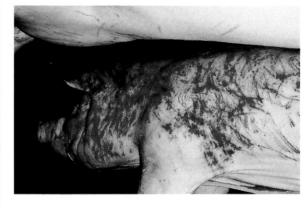

671 Fight wounds acquired in transit or in the lairage.

670 Wounds due to fighting after mixing Irrespective of housing and management objectives, sows on *loose* housing systems will have to be mixed sooner or later. In order to satisfy their natural inclination to establish a pecking order fighting will occur – sometimes resulting in the death of the modern hybrid sow.

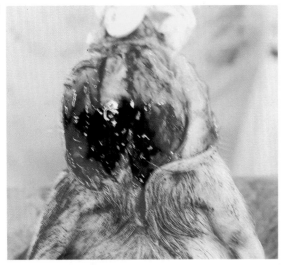

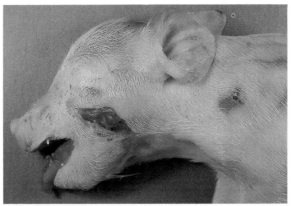

673 Savaging Death of newborn piglets due to savaging by dam (gilt).

672 Savaging Newborn piglet savaged by dam. Note injury over the cranium. The cause of savaging is not known but is likely to be associated with a young immature dam placed in a strange situation and severely stressed by farrowing and intensive housing. The prevalence is much higher in gilts than in older animals.

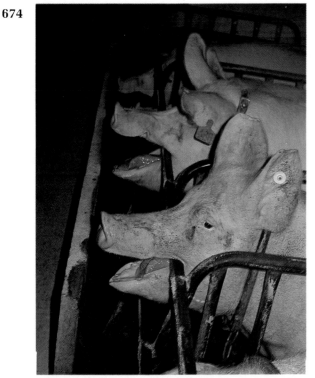

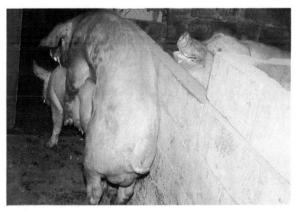

675 Sows refusing to stand to the boar It is now accepted that a sow in oestrus may have preference for a particular boar. In the above case, the sow would not stand to the boar to begin with but immediately stood when she happened to pass the other boar in the pen. She would have assumed that the boar in the pen was mating with her.

674 Bar biting in sows This may result in severe wear on the teeth (*see* **567**).

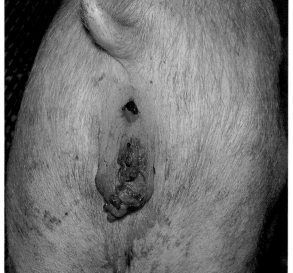

Vulva Biting – Sows

This vice has been noted since large groups of sows have been housed in strawed yards. Vulva biting has become a sporadic and very serious problem. Usually sows of parity four and above are involved, especially beyond 80 days of gestation. The injury received by the recipient can be catastrophic – even with one bite. One sow is usually responsible and during seconds (as opposed to minutes) can inflict an incredible amount of damage on her pen mates before she can be removed. These attacks appear to be unpremeditated. The following photographs exemplify some of the less serious injuries sustained by sows from their pen mates.

The disorder has also been noted in loose-housed sows fed at feeding stations, controlled by computer, where the sows have to reverse out after the completion of feeding.

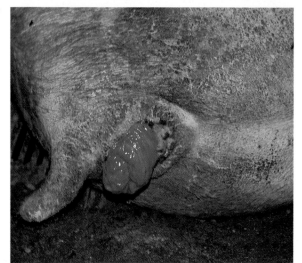

676 Vulva biting Note severe laceration of the vagina and relaxation of the anal sphincter.

677 Vulva biting Note the recto-vaginal fistula and rectal prolapse from severe damage to the perineal area.

678 Vulva biting Note severe damage to the anal sphincter.

679 Vulva biting Note haematoma of the damaged vaginal mucosa.

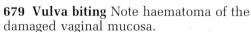

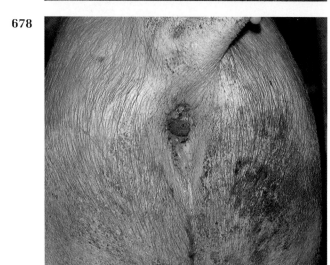

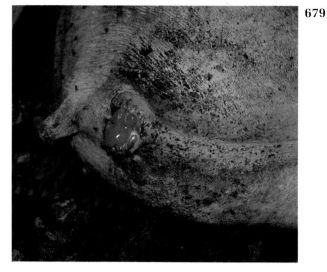

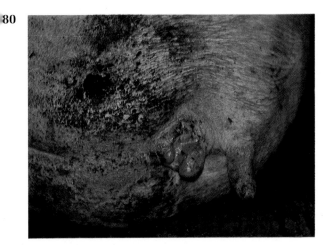

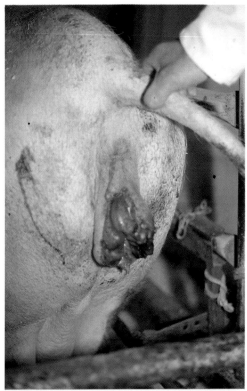

680 Vulva biting Newly-farrowed sow with severe distortion of the vulval aperture due to biting during gestation. Note the discharge due to chronic vaginitis.

681 Vulva biting Severe damage to the vulva of a sow (due to farrow) from biting. The vulva is often oedematous and easily damaged at this stage.

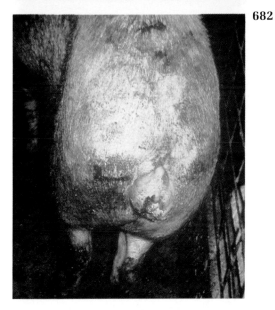

682 Vulva biting Vulval swelling at term associated with vulval biting.

Index

All references are to figure numbers